これからの
薬学英語

監修 野口ジュディー

著 天ヶ瀬葉子／神前陽子／スミス朋子／
玉巻欣子／堀 朋子／村木美紀子

English for Careers in Pharmaceutical Sciences

講談社

あらかじめご了承ください

・本書は全国の大学・専門学校で教材として使用されて
　いるため、練習問題の解答や日本語訳は付属していま
　せん。

執筆協力　Mariko Ono Guest（Pharm. D.）、Andrew Kirby（Ph. D.）
装丁　鮎川　廉（アユカワデザインアトリエ）

Foreword

Professional work requires professional communication. This is true regardless of whether the language is Japanese or English or another tongue. With the increasing global ties that connect peoples around the world today, English as a lingua franca for a professional is no longer an option but a requirement. This textbook was developed to help Japanese students of pharmaceutical sciences acquire the English language skills necessary for their future professions.

The ESP (English for specific purposes) approach of this textbook examines materials important for the profession. It tries to make students aware of the purpose, audience, information and language features of the genres, or types of text for example, over-the-counter interactions, Summary of Product Characteristics, online resources from the U.S. Food and Drug Administration as well as research articles.

This ESP approach is aimed at making students aware of genre features, how to examine them and how to master them. In the future, when they encounter new genres in their professions, this training should be useful for knowing how to deal with the new texts.

Judy Noguchi

本書を使われる先生方へ

　本書は、高学年向け薬学英語の教科書です。英語教育に関わる教員と薬学系教員・薬剤師との共同作業により作られたものです。薬学の専門知識のない英語教員と英語を教えた経験のない薬学系教員のどちらにも対応した教科書となっています。全てのレッスンを扱うには1年程度の期間が必要ですが、大学のシラバスに合わせ、Lessonを取捨選択して教えることが可能です。Lesson 1 - 5の医薬品情報やLesson 9のAbstractは英語学習に重きを置いて構成されています。また、Lesson 6, 7の服薬指導やLesson 10 - 13で扱う論文の本文は薬学の専門性が高いものとなっています。どのLessonも付属の教師用マニュアルを利用して指導できるようにしています。さらに、日本の学生が英語学習の中で苦手とする発音にも対応するべく音声資料を豊富に用意しました。ぜひ、ご活用ください。

まえがき

　専門分野の仕事は、専門的なコミュニケーションを通して進められます。これは、言語が日本語でも英語でも、また、他のどの言語でも当てはまることです。さらに、グローバル化によって世界中の人々が結び付けられている今日、専門性の高い仕事をする人々にとって、世界共通語としての英語の習得は、もはやオプションではなく必要要件となっています。この教科書は、日本の薬学生が、将来の職業に必要な英語力を身につけようとする際の助けとなるよう書かれたものです。

　この教科書では、専門分野における重要なジャンル（ジャンル＝専門的なコミュニケーションに必要な書き言葉および話し言葉のテキストの種類）の学習に、ESPアプローチで取り組みます。ESPとはEnglish for specific purposesの略語で、特定の目的のための英語（この教科書の場合は薬学のための英語）という意味です。みなさんは、各Lessonで提示される会話や文書が、どのような種類（ジャンル）に分類されるかを考えてください。会話は店頭でのやりとりなのか、入院時に交わされるものなのか、あるいは、文書は製品の概要を知らせるものなのか、政府機関からの勧告なのか、または研究論文なのか。ジャンルによってテキストの目的、オーディエンス、含まれる情報、そして言語的特徴が異なります。

　それらに注目しつつ、各Lessonの文書を読み解き、あるいは会話に参加することで、みなさんの「専門分野におけるジャンルとは何か、ジャンルにどのように取り組み、ジャンルをどのように使いこなすか」についての気づきを促すことがこの教科書の狙いです。ESPアプローチによる、この気づきは、みなさんが将来、薬学分野で仕事をする中で、新しいジャンルに出会ったときにも、きっと役立つことでしょう。

　なお、本書は薬学部の高学年の学生を対象としています。薬学部低学年の学生を対象とした本書の姉妹書「はじめての薬学英語」（講談社）が、薬学に関連する題材を広く扱っているのに対して、本書では、薬剤師としての業務に直接関わる題材（薬の添付文書、服薬指導など）や専門性の高い題材（プロトコール、原著論文など）を扱い、より実践的な内容になっています。

　この本の執筆にあたり、貴重な情報やご意見を賜りました同志社女子大学薬学部漆谷徹郎教授、髙橋玲教授、水川裕美子助教、川村暢幸助教、西村亜佐子助教、病態生理学研究室10期生の皆様、岡山大学病院薬剤部上嶋仁美薬剤師、School of Pharmacy, University of Southern California故Dr. Michael Wincor、Dr. Carla Blieden、Norwegian University of Science and Technology Mrs. Marylin Benzing に感謝申し上げます。また、立命館大学Dr. Nahla Hamouda、同志社女子大学現代社会学部Calum Adamson助教をはじめ音声教材作成にご協力いただきました先生方に御礼申し上げます。そして、終始適切にサポートを賜りました講談社サイエンティフィクの小笠原弘高氏に深謝いたします。最後になりましたが、現在アメリカで薬剤師として活躍されているDr. Mariko Ono Guest、イギリスの薬剤師Dr. Andrew Kirby (Xobaderm Ltd, Cardiff, UK)には教科書の企画の段階から原稿の校正までご協力いただきました。厚く御礼を申し上げ、感謝の意を表します。

2019年9月　著者一同

Contents

Foreword／本書を使われる先生方へ／まえがき iii

本書の内容構成と使い方 vi

Lesson 1 Drugstore Transaction: OTC Medicines 1
薬局での応対：外国人客にOTC薬を勧める

Lesson 2 Patient Information Leaflet (PIL) 7
患者向け医薬品情報書

Lesson 3 Summary of Product Characteristics (SmPC) 13
製品特性概要書

Lesson 4 Media Literacy for Pharmacists... 20
薬剤師のメディアリテラシー

Lesson 5 FDA website information on Clinical Trials.............................. 26
臨床試験に関するFDAのウェブサイト情報

Lesson 6 Medication Counseling 1 34
服薬指導(1)　初回面談・薬歴記載

Lesson 7 Medication Counseling 2 42
服薬指導(2)　処方提案・Drug Information (DI)

Lesson 8 Experiment Protocol.. 49
実験のプロトコール

Lesson 9 Research Article 1 : Title, Abstract 56
臨床試験の原著論文を読む(1)　表題と要旨

Lesson 10 Research Article 2 : Introduction 65
臨床試験の原著論文を読む(2)　序論

Lesson 11 Research Article 3 : Methods 73
臨床試験の原著論文を読む(3)　研究方法

Lesson 12 Research Article 4 : Results... 80
臨床試験の原著論文を読む(4)　結果

Lesson 13 Research Article 5 : Discussion, Comment 86
臨床試験の原著論文を読む(5)　考察

Appendix 1 イギリス英語・アメリカ英語の違い／2 おすすめの無料サイト／3 薬局や病院
での英語／4 英語文書・資料作成の基本／5 論文に出てくる表現集／6 発音に
注意すべき単語／7 Affixで覚える専門用語 90

v

本書の内容構成と使い方

　本書は、大きく分けて2部構成となっています。前半のLesson 1-7は薬剤師としての業務に直接関わる題材を扱っています。題材ごとに対患者コミュニケーションに必要な平易な表現と、医療従事者として身につけるべき専門的な表現の両方が学べるようになっています。後半のLesson 8-13では、実験のプロトコールと臨床系の原著論文を題材として、これらのジャンルの文書に特徴的かつ汎用性の高い表現を学び、同じジャンルの他の文書を読む際に適用できるように応用力の涵養を図ります。いずれにしても、専門文書の英文は、一文一文辞書を片手に全文を通して読むのではなく、目的を持って読むべき箇所を絞り込み、必要な情報を得ることを目指しましょう。本書ではそのコツを示しています。

【Lessonの内容】
Lesson 1：ドラッグストアで外国人客にOTC薬を勧める会話を学習します。用法・用量、使用上の注意など基本的なことを英語で説明する練習をしましょう。
Lesson 2-3：同じ製品の患者向け医薬品情報書と医療従事者用の製品特性概要書を扱っています。両者を比較し、薬剤師として知るべき専門的な情報が、英語でどのように表現されているか、また、得た情報をもとに外国人患者に説明するときに、情報をどのように取捨選択し、表現を患者向きに置き換えればよいのかを学びましょう。
Lesson 4：薬剤師が身につけるべきメディアリテラシーとして、英語による情報収集の仕方を紹介しています。外国人客・患者とコミュニケーションを取る際には、英語で情報収集したいものです。日本語で得た情報を誤解のないように英訳するには、皆さんが想像する以上に高度なスキルを必要とします。ぜひ、日本語を介さず、直接英語で情報収集するスキルを身につけてください。
Lesson 5：薬に対する反応が人種、民族などの違いによって異なる可能性を知りましょう。また、人種や民族の違いだけでなく、日本人とは異なる外国の文化、生活習慣や宗教などを理解して外国人客・患者と接することを心掛ける必要があります。
Lesson 6-7：初回面談、薬歴記載、処方提案など、様々なケースでの患者との会話をロールプレイの課題を通して学びます。外国人患者に平易な表現で説明できるようになりましょう。
Lesson 8：実験キットのプロトコールの読み方を学びます。実験のプロトコールは、日本語版が必ずあるとは限りません。実験方法でよく用いられる用語や表現を学習しましょう。
Lesson 9-13：臨床系の原著論文を扱います。特徴的な構造や頻出する表現を学びましょう。また、一文が長いものでも、主語と動詞を見つけて構造を分析できるように練習しましょう。

【音声の聞き方】
本書の紹介ページに、音声データが用意されています（収録箇所：各Lessonの ●)) の部分）。

紹介ページのアドレス
https://www.kspub.co.jp/book/detail/5172537.html

【各Lessonの構成】

1. タイトルの下には、各Lessonで扱うテキスト（文章や会話内容）の紹介がありますから、必ず読んでから学習を始めましょう。

2. Getting to know the genre

各Lessonで取り扱うジャンルの説明です。以下のPAILという4つのポイントに注目するとジャンルの特徴が理解でき、また同じジャンルに取り組む時に役立ちます。

Genre: 文書（または会話）の**タイプ・種類**

- ● Purpose: コミュニケーションの**目的**
- ● Audience *: どのような**受け手**（読み手）を対象に発信されたのか
- ● Information: どのような**情報**を伝えているのか
- ● Language features: どのような**言語的特徴**を持つか

*会話の場合Participants（参加者）となりますが、本書ではAudienceに統一しています。

3. Checking the terms

Lessonの内容理解や練習問題を解く時に必要な単語や表現を紹介します。病名や症状などの専門用語は、適宜本文中にも解説を入れています。

4. Reading the text

本文は、会話文、インターネットに掲載されている文章、医薬品情報、学術論文などがあります。出典があるものは原文を掲載しています。詳細に理解するべき部分もありますが、短時間で全体に目を通して必要な情報を探すことも大切なスキルです。

5. Exercise

問題を解いてジャンルについての理解を深め、頻出する表現や文法を学習しましょう。音声を聞いて答えを確認できるものもありますから、音読して適切に発音できるように練習しましょう。

6. Applying what you learned

Lessonで理解したことを発展・応用するための課題です。

7. Appendix (巻末)

参考資料をまとめたものです。練習問題を解く際などに活用しましょう。

【本書で使用する英語について】

　本書では、イギリスとアメリカの文書を掲載しているため、2国のspelling（綴り）と表現が用いられています。両者の違いはAppendixにまとめていますから参考にしてください。なお、Checking the termsには【英】もしくは【米】の表示と会話などの英文に≪British English≫、≪American English≫の表示があります。これは、綴り、表現、発音などがそれぞれイギリス式かアメリカ式かを示すものです。

　英語は母語としてだけではなく世界各地で公用語や共通語としても使われています。薬剤師として外国人とコミュニケーションする場合、非母語話者を対象として英語を用いる方が多いかもしれません。そのため、音声には、日本人、エジプト人など非母語話者の会話も含まれています。様々な英語に触れて、グローバルな英語を身につけましょう。

Lesson 1

Drugstore Transaction: OTC Medicines
薬局での応対：外国人客にOTC薬を勧める

　ドラッグストアは、保険や処方箋がなくても薬を購入でき、また便利な場所にあることも多いため、誰にとっても立ち寄りやすく、市販薬（OTC薬）を購入するため多くの外国人も訪れます。Lesson1では、

　①OTC薬を求めて薬局に来た外国人客に適切な薬を提供するため必要な情報を聞きとる

　②聞き取った情報を元に適切な薬を選び、安全に使用してもらえるよう服薬指導する

ことを学びます。

Getting to know the genre

Genre: OTC薬の販売時の会話

- **Purpose:** 　　　　　　使用者の症状に適したOTC薬を選び、正しく使用できるように指導する
- **Audience***: 　　　　　薬剤師・外国人客
- **Information:** 　　　　 来局者から聴取した情報、OTC薬の情報
- **Language features:** 専門知識を持たない人が理解できる平易な表現、疑問文、接客用語

*ここでは、Participants「本書の内容構成と使い方」参照

Checking the terms

active substance	有効成分	intraocular pressure	眼圧
belly button	へそ	OTC medicine（Over-The-Counter）	市販薬、OTC薬
currently	現在、目下		
diarrhea	下痢	persist	続く
dull pain	鈍い痛み	pit of the stomach	みぞおち
glaucoma	緑内障	sharp pain	鋭い痛み、さしこみ
heartburn	胸やけ	vomit	嘔吐する

1

Reading the text

腹痛を訴える30代の外国人男性がドラッグストアにOTC薬を求めて訪れました。症状や禁忌事項などを聞き取って、適したOTC薬を選び勧める必要があります。以下の会話文の意味を確認しながら、どのように必要な情報を聴取しているか確認しましょう。専門用語も出てきますから、音声を聞きながら正しく発音できるよう読む練習も行いましょう。　　　　　　　（ ⚫ Track01-1）

≪American English≫

Pharmacist: Hello. I'm a pharmacist. How may I help you?

Customer: Hi. I've had a stomachache for about a week.

Pharmacist: Where?

Customer: It's in the pit of my stomach, above the belly button.

5 Pharmacist: What is the pain like? A sharp pain or a dull pain?

Customer: Oh, it's a sharp pain.

Pharmacist: Do you have diarrhea, or did you vomit?
　　　　　　　　　　　　　　①　　　　　　　②

Customer: No runs, no throwing up. But I feel heartburn.

Pharmacist: I see. Before I recommend you a medicine, may I ask you about your general health?

10 Customer: Sure.

Pharmacist: Do you have glaucoma?

Customer: I don't think so. What is it?

Pharmacist: Have you ever been told by your doctor that your intraocular pressure is high? It's the
　　　　　　　　　　　　　　　　　　　　　　　　　　　　　　③
fluid pressure inside the eye.

15 Customer: Fluid pressure inside the eye? I have never had any problem with my eyes, so I don't
think so.

Pharmacist: Have you ever been told by your doctor that you should not take any particular type of
medicine?

Customer: Never. I have no allergy to any medicine as far as I know.

20 Pharmacist: Are you on any regular medication?

Customer: No, I'm not.

✏ Exercise 1

A. 下線部①～③の表現は会話の中で平易な言葉で表現されています。それぞれどの表現に言い換えられていますか？会話文中から探してみましょう。

	会話文中の平易な表現
① diarrhea	**1**
② vomit	**2**
③ intraocular pressure	**3**

2　*Lesson 1*

B. このドラッグストアには、この男性の症状に適した薬として、次の３つがあります。

選択肢（1）イラクナール錠

| 胃痛・腹痛・さしこみに | KDS 製薬 |

鎮痛鎮痙薬
イラクナール錠
Irakunal Tablets　　20 錠

胃痛・腹痛に　　**第２類医薬品**

イラクナール錠

［効能・効果］
胃痛、腹痛、さしこみ（疝痛、癪）、胃酸過多、胸やけ

［用法・用量］
成人（15 歳以上）1 回 1 錠、1 日 3 回を限度として、水またはぬるま湯で服用してください。服用間隔は 4 時間以上おいてください。

［成分］1 錠（1 回量）中
ブチルスコポラミン臭化物 10 mg
添加物：乳糖、白糖、マクロゴール、アラビアゴム、カルナウバロウ、サラシミツロウ、ステアリン酸 Mg、セラック、タルク、酸化チタン、トウモロコシデンプン、ラウリル硫酸 Na、酒石酸

（注意）
1. 次の人は服用しないでください。本剤または本剤の成分によりアレルギー症状を起こしたことがある人。
2. 服用後、乗物又は機械類の運転操作をしないでください。
3. 次の人は服用前に医師、薬剤師又は登録販売者に相談してください。(1) 医師の治療を受けている人。(2) 妊婦又は妊娠していると思われる人。(3) 高齢者。(4) 薬などによりアレルギー症状を起こしたことがある人。(5) 次の症状のある人。排尿困難。(6) 次の診断を受けた人。心臓病、緑内障
4. 服用に際しては、説明書をよく読んでください。
5. 直射日光の当たらない湿気の少ない涼しい所に保管してください。

選択肢（2）ファモブロックOD錠

| H₂ ブロッカー胃腸薬 | KDS 製薬 |

胃痛・もたれなどの胃の不快な症状に
ファモブロック OD 錠 10 mg
Famoblock OD

水なしでも服用できる口中溶解タイプ 6 錠

ファモブロック OD 錠　　**第１類医薬品**

［成分・分量］1錠中 ファモチジン 10 mg
添加物：リン酸水素 Ca、セルロース、乳糖、ヒドロキシプロピルセルロース、トウモロコシデンプン、無水ケイ酸、ステアリン酸 Ca、白糖、乳酸 Ca、マクロゴール、酸化チタン、タルク、カルナウバロウ

［効能・効果］胃痛、もたれ、胸やけ、むかつき
（本剤は H₂ ブロッカー薬を含んでいます）

［用法・用量］胃痛、もたれ、胸やけ、むかつきの症状があらわれた時、次の量を、口中で溶かして飲み込むか、水又はお湯で服用してください。

年齢	1回量	1日服用回数
成人 （15 歳以上、80 歳未満）	1 錠	2 回まで
小児（15 歳未満）	服用しないでください。	
高齢者（80 歳以上）		

＊服用後 8 時間以上たっても症状が治まらない場合は、もう1錠服用して下さい。
＊症状が治まった場合は、服用をやめて下さい。
＊3日間服用しても症状が改善しない場合は服用をやめて、医師又は薬剤師に相談してください。
＊2週間を超えて続けて服用しないでください。

注意
1. 次の人は服用しないで下さい。
(1) ファモチジンなどの H₂ ブロッカー薬によりアレルギー症状（例えば、発疹・発赤、かゆみ、のど・まぶた・口唇等の腫れ）を起こしたことがある人
(2) 医療機関で次の病気の治療や医薬品の投与を受けている人
血液の病気、腎臓・肝臓の病気、心臓の病気、胃・十二指腸の病気、喘息・リウマチ等の免疫系の病気、ステロイド剤、抗生物質、抗がん剤、アゾール系抗真菌剤
(3) 医師から赤血球が少ない（貧血）、血小板数が少ない（血が止まりにくい、血が出やすい）、白血球数が少ない等の血液異常を指摘されたことがある人。
(4) 小児（15 歳未満）及び高齢者（80 歳以上）
(5) 妊婦又は妊娠していると思われる人
2. 本剤を服用している間は、他の胃腸薬を服用しないで下さい。
3. 授乳中の人は本剤を服用しないか、本剤を服用する場合は授乳を避けて下さい。
4. 次の人は服用前に医師又は薬剤師に相談して下さい。
(1) 医師の治療を受けている又は他の医薬品を服用している人
(2) 薬などによりアレルギー症状を起こしたことがある人
(3) 高齢者（65 歳以上）
(4) 次の症状のある人
喉の痛み、吐気及び高熱、原因不明の体重減少、持続性の腹痛
5. 服用に際しては、説明文書をよくお読み下さい。
6. 直射日光の当たらない湿気の少ない涼しい所に保管して下さい。
7. 小児の手の届かない所に保管して下さい。
8. 表示の使用期限を過ぎた製品は使用しないで下さい。

選択肢（3）KDS漢方胃腸薬顆粒

KDS 漢方胃腸薬［顆粒］
KDS Kampo digestive medicine [granule]
安中散・芍薬甘草湯配合

胃もたれ
胸やけ
胃の不快感に

KDS 製薬株式会社　　24 包

KDS 漢方胃腸薬顆粒　**第２類医薬品**

［効能］胃のもたれ、胃部不快感、胃炎、胃痛、げっぷ、食欲不振、腹部膨満感、胸つかえ、胸やけ、胃酸過多、腹痛、吐き気

［用法・用量］次の量を食前又は食間に水又はぬるま湯で服用して下さい。

年齢	1回量	服用回数
成人（15 歳以上）	1 包	1 日 3 回
小児（5 歳以上 15 歳未満）	1/2 包	
5 歳未満	服用しないで下さい。	

安中散： 低下した胃腸機能を改善する胃腸薬
芍薬甘草湯： 胃の筋肉の緊張をほぐす胃の痛みを緩和する

［成分］

安中散（下記生薬の混合粉末）700 mg	
ケイヒ 200 mg	エンゴサク 150 mg
ボレイ 150 mg	ウイキョウ 75 mg
シュクシャ 50 mg	カンゾウ 50 mg
リュウコウ 25 mg	

芍薬甘草湯（下記生薬の抽出乾燥エキス末）170 mg	
シャクヤク 340 mg	カンゾウ 340 mg

添加物：バレイショデンプン、乳糖、セルロース、タルク

注意
1. 次の人は服用しないで下さい。
＊ 心臓病の診断を受けた人。
2. 次の人は服用前に医師、薬剤師又は登録販売員に相談して下さい。
＊ 医師の治療を受けている人
3. 服用に際しては、説明書をよく読んで下さい。
4. 直射日光の当たらない、湿気の少ない涼しい所に保管して下さい。
5. 小児の手の届かない所に保管して下さい。
6. 使用期限の過ぎた製品は、服用しないで下さい。

前のページの3つの薬から1つ選んで、実際に服薬指導の会話を作成します。まず、OTC薬の説明書は日本語で記載されているので、患者が後で参照できるように、重要な情報を以下のメモに英語でまとめましょう。成分名や効能の英語は調べましょう。

Commercial name of the medicine	**1**
Active substance(s)*	**2**
Directions	**3**
Warnings & precautions	**4**

*Active ingredient(s)ともいう

以下は選んだ薬を説明するモデル会話文です。上のメモや92ページのAppendixを参考にしながら、空欄に適切な表現を入れて完成させましょう。

Pharmacist: I recommend this medicine for your condition. The name of this medicine is (**5**   ) . The active substance (s) is / are (**6**   ) which (**7**   ) and will (**8**   ) your stomachache.

Customer: Oh, that's what I want. How do I take it?

5 Pharmacist: Take (**9**   ) . You may take it (**10**   ) .

Customer: Is this a common medicine? I mean, if I go to a pharmacy in my country, can I get the same stuff?

Pharmacist: I'm not certain if you can get the same one in your country, but it's likely that this medicine is / isn't available in your country as it is used in (**11**   )
10   countries.

Customer: I've never taken this medicine before. Is there anything I should be careful of?

Pharmacist: As you have never (**12**   ) an allergic reaction with medicines, you should be okay, but if you (**13**   ) rash, (**14**   ) in breathing or any other serious discomfort after taking this, stop taking and
15   (**15**   ) a physician or pharmacist. Please do not (**16**   ) .

Customer: Okay.

Pharmacist: I think it will help but if your symptoms persist or get worse, please contact me or visit a physician.

Customer: Thank you. I'll do so.

20 Pharmacist: Take care, thank you!

4   *Lesson 1*

Exercise 2

用法・用量の説明を練習しましょう。「(薬を) 飲む/服用する」という表現には、'drink'ではなく'take'を使うことに注意しましょう。説明する順番は、「1度に服用する量」⇒「回数」⇒「時間・タイミング」となります。服用回数や、服用時間などの表現は巻末のAppendix 3Aにまとめてありますので参考にして、以下の会話文を英語で表現してください。音声を聞いて、答え合わせをしましょう。

(🔊 **Track01-2**)

例：1回1錠、1日3回、毎食後飲んでください。

Take one tablet three times daily after every meal.

1 1回2錠、1日1回、朝食後に飲んでください。

2 1回1カプセル、1日2回、食間に飲んでください。

3 1回1包、1日1回、就寝前に飲んでください。

4 このシロップをお子さんに1回2目盛り分、6時間ごとに飲ませてください。

5 必要時に1錠飲んでもいいです。しかし、1日4回を超えて飲まないでください。

6 この薬は1回1カプセル、1日2回まで飲むことができますが、服用間隔を最低6時間あけてください。

7 この薬はチュアブル錠なので、よく噛んで服用してください。

8 1回1錠、1週間に1回、起床時にコップ1杯の水で服用し、服用後は30分間飲食せず、横にならないでください。毎週同じ曜日に必ず服用してください。

9 この湿布を患部に貼ってください。1日1回貼り替えてください。この湿布薬を貼った部位は衣服で覆い、直射日光を避けてください。

Applying what you learned

A. 以下の症状を訴える外国人客から話を詳しく聞き、市販されているOTC薬の中から適切な商品を選んで英語でロールプレイのシナリオを考えて練習しましょう。

1. 風邪の症状で来局。鼻水がたくさん出るが、咳は出ない。複数の成分を含む総合感冒薬を拒否し、「single-symptom formulaが欲しい」という。
2. 30代の母親と、身長が158 cmの10歳の男児が来局、アスピリンが欲しい。(誰がどのような症状で服用するのかは不明)。
3. 便秘を訴える若い女性が来局。妊娠の有無はわからない。
4. 花粉症で、鼻水と目のかゆみで困っている労働者風の男性が来局。工場で機械を扱っているので、眠くなりにくい薬が欲しい。
5. 日本滞在中に足首を捻挫した60代女性が来局。捻挫に効く外用薬があると聞いたが、今までに使ったことがなく、どのような薬なのか、どう使うのかを知りたい。
6. 乗り物酔いで困っている5歳の子供をつれて母親が来局。何か薬が欲しいが、その子供は錠剤が飲めない。

B. 薬には副作用がたくさんあります。薬の副作用としてどのようなものが思い浮かびますか？グループやペアで代表的な副作用をできるだけたくさん書き出して、英語で何というか調べましょう。以下の図はFDAのウェブサイトに掲載されているものです。参考にしてみましょう。

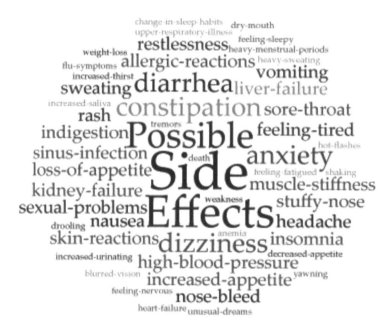

https://www.fda.gov/drugs/drug-information-consumers/finding-and-learning-about-side-effects-adverse-reactions

Lesson 2

Patient Information Leaflet (PIL)
患者向け医薬品情報書

　自分が飲んでいる薬について知りたいと思った時、患者は薬剤師に直接相談するか、薬と共に手渡された医薬品情報提供書を参照することができますが、最近では患者自身がインターネットで詳しい情報を検索することも少なくありません。医療情報には多くの専門用語が含まれますが、専門知識をもたない人にもわかるように平易な言葉で書かれた情報も提供されています。医療用医薬品について、日本では患者向医薬品ガイド*やくすりのしおり**などが用意されています。イギリスでは、Medicines and Healthcare products Regulatory Agency（MHRA: 英国医薬品医療製品規制庁）がPatient Information Leaflet（PIL: 医薬品情報書）を出しています。Lesson 2では高血圧治療薬アムロジピンのPILを紹介します。

*患者向医薬品ガイド(医薬品医療機器総合機構)：https://www.pmda.go.jp/safety/info-services/drugs/items-information/guide-for-patients/0001.html
**くすりのしおり(くすりの適正使用協議会)：http://www.rad-ar.or.jp/siori/　（英語版もあり）

▷ Getting to know the genre

Genre: 患者向け医薬品情報書

- **Purpose:**　　　　　　処方薬を安全に使用してもらう
- **Audience:**　　　　　　薬を処方された患者
- **Information:**　　　　　適応症、用法・用量、注意事項など
- **Language features:**　命令文、should の使用、箇条書き

Checking the terms

adolescent	青少年 ※10-19歳 WHOによる定義
blister pack	PTP(press through package)包装
breast-feeding	授乳
casualty department[英]	救命救急部
clammy	冷や汗が出た
dose	薬の一回量
elderly	高齢者
expiry	使用期限
follow	従う、守る
halves	halfの複数形

immediately	直ちに
leaflet	（通常1枚の）説明書
obtain	得る
overdose	過量摂取
pregnancy	妊娠
prescribe	処方する
prescription	処方（箋）
side effect	副作用
store	保管する
strength	（主成分の）含有量、力価

Reading the text

CP.AML.JNT.T.SH.V1P1

PATIENT INFORMATION LEAFLET

AMLODIPINE 5mg AND 10mg TABLETS

Read all of this leaflet carefully before you start taking this medicine because it contains important information for you.
- Keep this leaflet. You may need to read it again.
- If you have any more questions, please ask your doctor or your pharmacist.
- This medicine has been prescribed for you personally and you should not pass it on to anyone else. It may harm them, even if their symptoms are the same as yours.
- If any of the side effects get serious, or if you notice any side effects that are not listed in the leaflet, please tell your doctor or pharmacist.

In this leaflet:
1. What Amlodipine Tablets are and what they are used for
2. What you need to know before you take Amlodipine Tablets
3. How to take Amlodipine Tablets
4. Possible side effects
5. How to store Amlodipine Tablets
6. Contents of the pack and other information

The name of your medicine is Amlodipine 5mg Tablets or Amlodipine 10mg Tablets. We refer to them as Amlodipine Tablets or amlodipine throughout this leaflet.

1. WHAT AMLODIPINE TABLETS ARE AND WHAT THEY ARE USED FOR

Amlodipine Tablets contain the active substance amlodipine which belongs to a group of medicines called calcium antagonists.

Amlodipine Tablets may be used to treat:
- high blood pressure (hypertension); and
- a certain type of chest pain called angina, a rare form of which is Prinzmetal's or variant angina.

In patients with high blood pressure, these medicines work by relaxing blood vessels, so that blood passes through them more easily. In patients with angina, amlodipine works by improving blood supply to the heart muscle which then receives more oxygen and as a result chest pain is prevented. Amlodipine Tablets do not immediately relieve chest pain caused by angina.

2. WHAT YOU NEED TO KNOW BEFORE YOU TAKE AMLODIPINE TABLETS

Do not take Amlodipine Tablets if you:
- have ever had an allergic reaction to amlodipine or any of the ingredients in the tablet listed in section 6, or to any other calcium antagonist. An allergic reaction may include a rash, itching, difficulty breathing or swelling of the face, lips, throat or tongue;
- have very low blood pressure (hypotension) so that you feel faint or dizzy;
- have cardiogenic shock (a condition where your heart cannot pump enough blood for your body's needs);
- have heart failure due to a heart attack;
- have narrowing of the heart valve of the aorta (aortic stenosis).

Take special care with Amlodipine Tablets
You should inform your doctor if you have or have had any of the following conditions:
- Recent heart attack;
- Heart failure;
- Liver disease;
- You are elderly and your dose needs to be increased;
- Severe increase in blood pressure (Hypertensive crisis).

Use in children and adolescents
Amlodipine has not been studied in children under the age of 6 years. Amlodipine should only be used for hypertension in children and adolescents from 6 years to 17 years of age (see section 3).
For more information, talk to your doctor.

Taking other medicines and Amlodipine
Please tell your doctor or pharmacist if you are taking or have recently taken other medicines, including medicines obtained without a prescription.

Amlodipine may affect or be affected by other medicines, such as:
- diltiazem, verapamil (heart medicines)
- ketoconazole, itraconazole (antifungal medicines used to treat thrush and ringworm)
- ritonavir, indinavir, nelfinavir (antivirals used in treatment of HIV infections)
- rifampicin, erythromycin, clarithromycin (antibiotics)
- St John's wort (a herbal remedy for mild depression)
- dantrolene (infusion for severe body temperature abnormalities)
- simvastatin (a drug used to control elevated cholesterol)

Amlodipine may lower your blood pressure even more if you are already taking other medicines to treat your high blood pressure.

If you see another doctor or go into hospital for any reason, tell them that you are taking Amlodipine Tablets.

Taking Amlodipine Tablets with food and drink
You should not drink grapefruit juice or eat grapefruit while taking this medicine. Grapefruit and grapefruit juice can lead to an increase in the blood levels of amlodipine, which can cause an unpredictable increase in its blood pressure lowering effect.

Pregnancy
The safety of amlodipine in human pregnancy has not been established. If you think you might be pregnant, or are planning to get pregnant, you must tell your doctor before you take Amlodipine Tablets.

Breast-feeding
It is not known whether amlodipine is passed into breast milk. If you are breast-feeding or about to start breast-feeding you must tell your doctor before taking Amlodipine Tablets.

Ask your doctor or pharmacist for advice before taking any medicine.

Driving and using machines
Taking Amlodipine Tablets may affect your ability to drive or use machinery because amlodipine could cause side effects such as dizziness, headaches, nausea or tiredness, all of which could affect your ability to concentrate.

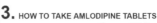

3. HOW TO TAKE AMLODIPINE TABLETS

Swallow these tablets with a glass of water at the same time each day. You can take the tablets either before or after meals.
Follow your doctor's instructions. Check the pharmacy label to see how many tablets to take and how often to take them. If you are still not sure, ask your pharmacist or doctor. The usual doses are described below.

Adults
One 5mg tablet once a day. Your doctor may increase the dose to one 10mg tablet once a day.

Children and adolescents
For children and adolescents, (6-17 years old), the recommended usual starting dose is 2.5mg a day. The maximum recommended dose is 5mg a day. Amlodipine 2.5mg is not currently available and the 2.5mg dose cannot be obtained with Amlodipine 5mg or 10mg Tablets as these tablets are not manufactured to break into two equal halves.

Elderly
As for adults (one 5mg tablet a day). Your doctor will closely monitor your response to any increase in the dose.

Patients with liver disease
Your doctor may give you a different dose to normal.

If you take more Amlodipine Tablets than you should
If you (or someone else) swallow a lot of tablets all together, or if you think a child has swallowed any of the tablets, contact your nearest hospital casualty department or your doctor immediately. Take your medication and the packaging with you to the doctor or casualty department. If you have

8 Lesson 2

taken an overdose, you may appear flushed (your skin will look red), or you may feel dizzy or faint. If blood pressure drop is severe enough shock can occur. Your skin could feel cool or clammy and you could lose consciousness.

If you forget to take Amlodipine Tablets
If you forget to take a tablet, take one as soon as you remember, unless it is nearly time to take the next one. Never take two doses together. Take the remaining doses at the correct time.

If you stop taking Amlodipine Tablets
Take this medicine for as long as your doctor tells you to, as you may become unwell if you stop.

4. POSSIBLE SIDE EFFECTS

Like all medicines, Amlodipine Tablets can cause side effects, although not everybody gets them.
If any of the following reactions happen, stop taking Amlodipine Tablets and tell your doctor immediately or contact the casualty department at your nearest hospital:
• swelling of the eyelids, face, lips
• swelling of the tongue and throat which causes great difficulty breathing
• sudden wheeziness, chest pain, difficulty breathing or swallowing
• severe skin reactions including itching, rash, peeling of the skin and extensive reddening, blistering or swelling of the skin, inflammation of mucous membranes (Stevens-Johnson syndrome) or other allergic reactions
• heart attack, abnormal heart beat,
• inflamed pancreas which can cause severe abdominal and back pain accompanied with feeling very unwell.

Other known side effects are as follows. Tell your doctor if you notice or are worried by any of the side effects listed.

Common (affects 1 to 10 users in 100)
• headache, drowsiness, dizziness (especially at the start of treatment)
• flushing of the face and feeling hot
• feeling sick, stomach ache
• tiredness
• palpitations (irregular or forceful heart beat)
• swollen ankles

Uncommon (affects 1 to 10 users in 1,000)
• enlargement or discomfort of the breasts in men
• a general feeling of being unwell, weakness
• change in taste, dry mouth
• involuntary shakiness, numbness, tingling or pins and needles
• loss of pain sensation
• increased sweating
• sight problems, double vision
• problems sleeping, irritability, depression, mood changes
• fainting
• low blood pressure
• sneezing/runny nose caused by inflammation of the lining of the nose (rhinitis)
• being sick, diarrhoea, constipation, indigestion
• itchy skin, red patches on skin, skin discolouration
• hair loss
• muscle cramps, back, muscle or joint pain
• passing urine more often, night time urinating
• inability to obtain an erection
• weight loss or gain
• ringing in the ears

Rare (affects 1 to 10 users in 10,000)
• confusion

Very rare (affects less than 1 user in 10,000)
• decreased numbers of white blood cells, decrease in blood platelets which may result in unusual bruising or easy bleeding
• raised blood sugar levels (hyperglycaemia)
• problems feeling through fingers and toes due to nerve problems (peripheral neuropathy)
• inflammation of the blood vessels, often with skin rash
• abdominal bloating (gastritis)
• cough
• swollen gums
• raised liver enzymes (detected in a blood test), yellowing of the skin or whites of the eyes (jaundice, hepatitis)
• increased muscle tension
• sensitivity to light
• disorders combining rigidity, tremor and/or movement disorders

Tell your doctor or pharmacist if you notice any other effects not listed.

Reporting of side effects
If you get any side effects, talk to your doctor or pharmacist. This includes any possible side effects not listed in this leaflet. You can also report side effects directly via the Yellow Card Scheme, Website: www.mhra.gov.uk/yellowcard. By reporting side effects you can help provide more information on the safety of this medicine.

5. HOW TO STORE AMLODIPINE TABLETS

Do not use the tablets after the end of the expiry month (use-by date) shown on the product packaging.
Do not store the tablets above 30°C.
Store in the original package.

KEEP THIS MEDICINE OUT OF THE SIGHT AND REACH OF CHILDREN

Medicines should not be disposed of via wastewater or household waste. Ask your pharmacist how to dispose of medicines no longer required. These measures will help to protect the environment.

6. CONTENTS OF THE PACK AND OTHER INFORMATION

What Amlodipine Tablets contain
• The active substance is amlodipine as amlodipine mesilate monohydrate.
  Each tablet contains 5mg or 10mg of amlodipine.
• The other ingredients are microcrystalline cellulose, anhydrous calcium hydrogen phosphate, sodium starch glycolate type A and magnesium stearate.

What Amlodipine Tablets look like and the contents of the pack
Amlodipine Tablets are white to off-white, round and biconvex and come in two strengths – 5mg and 10mg.
The 5mg tablets have the number '5' embossed on one side and the 10mg tablets have the number '10' embossed on one side, together with a breakline.
Amlodipine Tablets are available in blister packs containing 10, 14, 20, 28, 30, 50, 98, 100 or 200 tablets.
Not all pack sizes may be marketed.

Marketing authorisation holder:
Athlone Pharmaceuticals Limited, Ballymurray, Co. Roscommon, Ireland.

Manufacturer responsible for batch release:
Kent Pharmaceuticals Limited, Crowbridge Road, Ashford, Kent, TN24 0GR, U.K.
Kent Pharmaceuticals Limited, Repton Road, Measham, DE12 7DT, U.K.

This medicinal product is authorised in the member states of the EEA under the following names.

United Kingdom:	Amlodipine 5mg Tablets
	Amlodipine 10mg Tablets
Ireland:	Amlotan 5mg Tablets
	Amlotan 10mg Tablets

This leaflet was last revised in July 2014.

PMLLDPA01
DDDPALL00ABGIE

CP.AML.JNT.T.SH.V1P1

Exercise 1

PILには患者が医薬品を適正に使用するために知っておくべきさまざまな情報が1枚に詰め込まれています。

A. 全体に目を通し、以下の情報を探しましょう。

薬の名称	**1**
薬の剤型	**2**
薬を製造した製薬会社	**3**
この製薬会社が所在する国名	**4**
この*PILの最終改訂日	**5**

＊PILは、新たな情報が入手されると改訂されるため、最終改訂日を確認することが重要です。

B. 以下の**1**～**6**はこのPILのHeading（見出し）です。多くの情報がどのように整理されているか確認し、日本の医薬品添付文書（医療従事者用）の表現と対応させて線で結びましょう。

1 What Amlodipine Tablets are and what they are used for ・　　　　　・ 用法・用量

2 What you need to know before you take Amlodipine Tablets ・　　　　　・ 組成・性状

3 How to take Amlodipine Tablets ・　　　　　・ 効能・効果

4 Possible side effects ・　　　　　・ 副作用

5 How to store Amlodipine Tablets ・　　　　　・ 使用上の注意

6 Contents of the pack and other information ・　　　　　・ 貯法

Exercise 2

A. 患者が以下の事柄について知りたいとき、PILの6つのSectionのうちどれを読むべきですか？　その番号を記入してください。また、これらの質問に答えるために読むべき箇所に線をひきましょう。

1 What kind of illness is this medicine used for?　　　　　　Section No. (　　)

2 What kinds of side effects should I be careful of?　　　　　Section No. (　　)

3 What kinds of ingredients are contained in this tablet?　　　Section No. (　　)

4 Is there any food that cannot be taken together with this medicine?

Section No. (　　)

5 How should I keep this medicine at home?　　　　　　　　Section No. (　　)

B. PILの内容を、患者目線でもう少し詳しく読んでみましょう。詳しい情報を探すときは、各Section内の太字で書かれたSubheading（小見出し）に注目しましょう。次の患者の疑問に答える情報は、どこに含まれていますか？　Sectionの番号を示していますのでそのSection内で参照すべきSubheadingを（　　　）に書き入れましょう。

1 "I didn't tell my doctor that I have been taking St John's wort. Why can't I take this medicine and St John's wort together?"
Section 2　Subheading (　　　　　　　　　　　　　　　　　　　　　　　　　　　)

2 "I am planning to have a baby. Is it safe to take this medicine while I am trying?"
Section 2　Subheading (　　　　　　　　　　　　　　　　　　　　　　　　　　　)

3 "I took more of this medicine than I should have. Could this affect me badly? What should I do?"
Section 3　Subheading (　　　　　　　　　　　　　　　　　　　　　　　　　　　)

4 "I forgot to take this medicine yesterday. Should I take two doses today?"
Section 3　Subheading (　　　　　　　　　　　　　　　　　　　　　　　　　　　)

5 "I get a headache after taking this medicine. Is it a side effect? "
Section 4　Subheading (　　　　　　　　　　　　　　　　　　　　　　　　　　　)

C. PILには、薬局での服薬指導時に応用できる表現も含まれています。PILにある表現を参考にして、以下の日本語を英語にして、音声を聞いて確認しましょう。　　　（ Track02-1）

1 この薬はあなたに処方されたもので、他人に手渡してはいけません。

2 この薬を服用した後に体調が悪くなったら医師または薬剤師に連絡してください。

3 薬は子供の目につかない手の届かないところで保管してください。

4 授乳中の方は、この薬を服用する前に医師に伝えてください。

5 この薬を服用すると、車の運転や機械の操作に影響がでるかもしれません。

11

D. Section 4の Possible Side Effectsでは、発生頻度ごとに副作用がまとめられています。以下の表の空欄を埋めましょう。

Common 頻度：(**1**)%〜(**2**)%		Uncommon 頻度：(**3**)%〜(**4**)%	
英語	日本語	英語	日本語
5	頭痛	**12**	脱力感
drowsiness	**6**	**13**	味覚異常
dizziness	**7**	dry mouth	**14**
flushing	**8**	involuntary shakiness	不随意の震え
9	悪心	numbness	**15**
10	胃痛、腹痛	sweating	**16**
tiredness	**11**	double vision	複視
swollen ankles	足首の腫れ	**17**	うつ状態

➡ Applying what you learned

以下の薬剤（処方薬）のPILをダウンロードして、その内容を説明するスライドを作って発表しましょう（巻末のAppendix 4 B参照）。

アスピリン	クラリスロマイシン	オメプラゾール	カンデサルタン
アセトアミノフェン（パラセタモール*）	カルボシステイン	メトホルミン	シンバスタチン
イトラコナゾール	ニフェジピン	アロプリノール	メトトレキサート

*日本や北米でアセトアミノフェンと呼ばれる薬は、多くの国でパラセタモールと呼ばれています。このように一般名が複数ある薬も存在します。

※発表のヒント

①選んだ薬剤の英語表記を確認する。

② a) 効能・効果、b) 用法・用量、c) 使用上の注意、d) 副作用情報について簡潔に説明する。

③患者役と薬剤師役の会話のロールプレイをする

④引用した情報の出典を明示する（ダウンロードしたPILのURLなど）

Lesson 3

Summary of Product Characteristics (SmPC)
製品特性概要書

　日本では、医薬品の箱に必ずその添付文書が同梱されており、医療従事者は信頼できる医薬品の詳細な情報をこの文書から得ます。欧州でこの文書にあたるのが、Summary of Product Characteristics（SmPC: 製品特性概要書または欧州製品概要）で、European Medicines Agency（EMA: 欧州医薬品庁）が発行しています。これらの文書は、副作用や適応症の拡大など新しい情報が発表されたらその都度、内容が更新されます。記載される内容が同じでも、Lesson 2で取り扱った患者など一般の人を対象としたPILと医療従事者用のSmPCでは言葉遣いや表現、内容にどのような違いがあるか注目しましょう。

※　海外の添付文書情報は、日本医薬情報センターのウェブサイトにリンクがあるので参考にしてください。
　　https://www.japic.or.jp/di/navi.php?cid=1

Getting to know the genre

Genre:SmPC: 製品特性概要書（欧州製品概要）
- **Purpose:** 　　　患者の安全を確保し、処方薬の適正使用を図るために情報を提供する
- **Audience:** 　　医療従事者
- **Information:** 　　適応症、用法・用量、禁忌事項、作用機序、代謝機構など
- **Language features:** 専門用語、見出し、箇条書き、図表

Checking the terms

administration	投与	paediatric[英]	小児の
biconvex	両凸の	posology	薬量学（用法・用量）
concomitant	併用の	precaution	事前注意
contraindication	禁忌	qualitative	質的な
dosage	服用量	quantitative	量的な
efficacy	有効性	refractory	難治性の
embossed	型が押された	regimen	レジメン、投与計画
excipient	添加物	renal impairment	腎障害
fertility	生殖能力	therapeutic indication	適応症
foetus[英]	胎児		
hepatic impairment	肝障害	tolerate	耐える、忍容する
monotherapy	単剤療法	warning	警告

13

Reading the text

以下は、Amlodipine 10 mg Tablet の SmPC の抜粋です。全文は electronic Medicines Compendium（eMC）のウェブサイトを参照してください。

https://www.medicines.org.uk/emc/product/2114/smpc

Amlodipine 10 mg Tablet SmPC

Kent Pharmaceuticals Ltd
Active ingredient   amlodipine mesilate monohydrate
Legal Category   POM: Prescription only medicine

5 **1. Name of the medicinal product**
Amlodipine 10 mg tablet

2. Qualitative and quantitative composition
Each tablet contains 10 mg amlodipine (as amlodipine mesilate monohydrate).
For excipients, see 6.1.

10 **3. Pharmaceutical form**
Tablet
The tablets are white to off-white, round biconvex and embossed with "10" on one side.

4. Clinical particulars

4.1 Therapeutic indications
15 Hypertension
Chronic stable angina pectoris
Vasospastic (Prinzmetal's) angina
4.2 Posology and method of administration
Posology
20 *Adults*
For both hypertension and angina the usual initial dose is 5 mg amlodipine once daily which may be increased to a maximum dose of 10 mg depending on the individual patient's response.
In hypertensive patients, amlodipine has been used in combination with a thiazide diuretic, alpha blocker, beta blocker, or an angiotensin converting enzyme inhibitor. For angina, amlodipine may be used as monotherapy or in combination with other
25 antianginal medicinal products in patients with angina that is refractory to nitrates and/or to adequate doses of beta blockers.
No dose adjustment of amlodipine is required upon concomitant administration of thiazide diuretics, beta blockers, and angiotensin-converting enzyme inhibitors.
Special populations
Elderly
30 Amlodipine used at similar doses in elderly or younger patients is equally well tolerated. Normal dosage regimens are recommended in the elderly, but increase of the dosage should take place with care (see sections 4.4 and 5.2).
Renal impairment
Changes in amlodipine plasma concentrations are not correlated with degree of renal impairment, therefore the normal dosage is recommended. Amlodipine is not dialysable.
35 *Hepatic impairment*
Dosage recommendations have not been established in patients with mild to moderate hepatic impairment; therefore dose selection should be cautious and should start at the lower end of the dosing range (see sections 4.4 and 5.2). The pharmacokinetics of amlodipine have not been studied in severe hepatic impairment. Amlodipine should be initiated at the lowest dose and titrated slowly in patients with severe hepatic impairment.
40 *Paediatric population*
Children and adolescents with hypertension from 6 years to 17 years of age.
The recommended antihypertensive oral dose in paediatric patients aged 6-17 years is 2.5 mg once daily as a starting dose, up-titrated to 5 mg once daily if blood pressure goal is not achieved after 4 weeks. Doses in excess of 5 mg daily have not been studied in paediatric patients (see sections 5.1 and 5.2).
45 Doses of amlodipine 2.5 mg are not possible with this medicinal product.
Children under 6 years old
No data are available.
Method of administration
Tablet for oral administration.
50 **4.3 Contraindications**
Amlodipine is contra-indicated in patients with:
• Severe hypotension

14   *Lesson 3*

- shock (including cardiogenic shock)
- hypersensitivity to dihydropyridine derivatives, amlodipine or any of the excipients.
55 • haemodynamically unstable heart failure after acute myocardial infarction
- obstruction of the outflow-tract of the left ventricle (e.g. high grade aortic stenosis)

4.4 Special warnings and precautions for use

The safety and efficacy of amlodipine in hypertensive crisis has not been established.

Patients with cardiac failure

60 Patients with cardiac failure should be treated with caution. In a long-term, placebo controlled study in patients with severe heart failure (NYHA class III and IV) the reported incidence of pulmonary oedema was higher in the amlodipine treated group than in the placebo group (see section 5.1).

Calcium channel blockers, including amlodipine, should be used with caution in patients with congestive heart failure, as they may increase the risk of future cardiovascular events and mortality.

65 *Use in patients with impaired hepatic function*

The half life of amlodipine is prolonged and AUC values are higher in patients with impaired liver function; dosage recommendations have not been established. Amlodipine should therefore be initiated at the lower end of the dosing range and caution should be used, both on initial treatment and when increasing the dose. Slow dose titration and careful monitoring may be required in patients with severe hepatic impairment

70 *Use in elderly patients*

In the elderly, increase of the dosage should take place with care (see sections 4.2 and 5.2).

Use in renal failure

Amlodipine may be used in such patients at normal doses. Changes in amlodipine plasma concentrations are not correlated with degree of renal impairment. Amlodipine is not dialysable.

75 **4.5 Interaction with other medicinal products and other forms of interaction**

Effects of other medicinal products on amlodipine

CYP3A4 inhibitors: Concomitant use of amlodipine with strong or moderate CYP3A4 inhibitors (protease inhibitors, azole antifungals, macrolides like erythromycin or clarithromycin, verapamil or diltiazem) may give rise to significant increase in amlodipine exposure. The clinical translation of these PK variations may be more pronounced in the elderly. Clinical monitoring and
80 dose adjustment may thus be required.

CYP3A4 inducers: There is no data available regarding the effect of CYP3A4 inducers on amlodipine. The concomitant use of CYP3A4 inducers (e.g., rifampicin, hypericum perforatum) may give a lower plasma concentration of amlodipine. Amlodipine should be used with caution together with CYP3A4 inducers.

Administration of amlodipine with grapefruit or grapefruit juice is not recommended as bioavailability may be increased in some
85 patients resulting in increased blood pressure lowering effects.

Dantrolene (infusion): In animals, lethal ventricular fibrillation and cardiovascular collapse are observed in association with hyperkalaemia after administration of verapamil and intravenous dantrolene. Due to risk of hyperkalaemia, it is recommended that the co-administration of calcium channel blockers such as amlodipine be avoided in patients susceptible to malignant hyperthermia and in the management of malignant hyperthermia.

90 *Effects of amlodipine on other medicinal products*

The blood pressure lowering effects of amlodipine adds to the blood pressure-lowering effects of other medicinal products with antihypertensive properties.

In clinical interaction studies, amlodipine did not affect the pharmacokinetics of atorvastatin, digoxin, warfarin or cyclosporin.

Simvastatin: Co-administration of multiple doses of 10 mg of amlodipine with 80 mg simvastatin resulted in a 77% increase in
95 exposure to simvastatin compared to simvastatin alone. Limit the dose of simvastatin in patients on amlodipine to 20 mg daily.

4.6 Fertility, pregnancy and lactation

Pregnancy

The safety of amlodipine in human pregnancy has not been established.

In animal studies, reproductive toxicity was observed at high doses (see section 5.3).

100 Use in pregnancy is only recommended when there is no safer alternative and when the disease itself carries greater risk for the mother and foetus.

Breast-feeding It is not known whether amlodipine is excreted in breast milk.

A decision on whether to continue/discontinue breast-feeding or to continue/discontinue therapy with amlodipine should be made taking into account the benefit of breast-feeding to the child and the benefit of amlodipine therapy to the woman.

105 Fertility

Reversible biochemical changes in the head of spermatozoa have been reported in some patients treated by calcium channel blockers. Clinical data are insufficient regarding the potential effect of amlodipine on fertility. In one rat study, adverse effects were found on male fertility (see section 5.3).

Exercise 1

各国添付文書におけるSectionのHeading（見出し）の対応を確認しましょう。以下の表には、Lesson 2で見たPILと、アメリカおよび日本の添付文書のSection Headingの一部があらかじめ記載されています。ここに、SmPCのHeadingを当てはめましょう。

英欧日米　添付文書表現の比較（抜粋）

英（UK）	欧（EU）	日（Japan）	米（USA）
Patient Information Leaflet (PIL)	Summary of Product Characteristics (SmPC)	医薬品添付文書	Prescribing Information (PI)*
患者、一般の人用	医療従事者用	医療従事者用	医療従事者用
What Amlodipine tablets are used for	**1**	効能・効果	Indications and Usage
How to take Amlodipine tablets	**2**	用法・用量	Dosage and Administration
Do not take Amlodipine tablets if you…	**3**	禁忌	Contraindications
Possible Side Effects	Undesirable effects	副作用	Adverse Reactions
Taking other medicines and Amlodipine	**4**	相互作用	Drug Interactions
Take special care with Amlodipine tablets	Special warnings and precautions for use	●警告 ●使用上の注意	Warnings and Precautions

*医薬品の添付文書は、米国ではPrescribing Informationと表示されるほか、LabelやPackage Insert（医薬品の包装に挿入されているものという意味）とよばれることもあります。

Exercise 2

A. Section 4.1 Therapeutic indicationsを読みましょう。Therapeutic indicationsとは医薬品の適応症の事で、その医薬品をどのような病気や病態に使用するのかを示します。SmPCに記載されている適応症の表現と、Lesson 2のPILの表現を比較してみましょう。

SmPCの表現	PILの表現
1. Hypertension	**1**
2. Chronic stable angina pectoris Vasospastic (Prinzmetal's) angina	**2**

16　*Lesson 3*

B. Section 4.2 Posology and method of administrationを読みましょう。

1. 成人に対するアムロジピンの用法・用量についての記述も、SmPCとPILでは以下のように
   表現が違います。

SmPCの表現	PILの表現
For both hypertension and angina the usual initial dose is 5 mg amlodipine once daily which may be increased to a maximum dose of 10 mg depending on the individual patient's response.	One 5 mg tablet once a day. Your doctor may increase the dose to one 10 mg tablet once a day.

SmPCに記載されているアムロジピンの用法用量を日本語で説明しましょう。

1

2. Special populationと呼ばれる患者はどのような患者ですか？　下の表にまとめましょう。

SmPCに記載されたspecial population	日本語訳
2	7
3	8
4	9
5	10
6	11

C. Section 4.3 Contraindicationsに書かれているアムロジピンの禁忌5項目を日本語で書き
ましょう。

Severe hypotension	1
Shock (including cardiogenic shock)	2
Hypersensitivity to dihydropyridine derivatives, amlodipine or any of the excipients	3
Haemodynamically unstable heart failure after acute myocardial infarction	4
Obstruction of the outflow-tract of the left ventricle (e.g. high grade aortic stenosis)	5

D. Section 4.5 Interaction with other medicinal products and other forms of interactionに
記載されているアムロジピン服用中のグレープフルーツの摂取について詳しく読みましょう。
下の表の左側はPILでグレープフルーツの摂取について言及されている部分を抜粋したもの
です。下線部の内容が、SmPCではどのように表現されているか比較して、（　　　）に英語
を書き入れましょう。

PIL	SmPC
drink grapefruit juice or eat grapefruit while <u>taking</u> this medicine	(**1**) of amlodipine with grapefruit or grapefruit juice
can lead to an increase in <u>the blood levels of</u> amlodipine	(**2**) may be increased in some patients
<u>can cause</u> an unpredictable increase in its blood pressure lowering effect	(**3**) increased blood pressure lowering effects

E. Section 4.6 Fertility, pregnancy and lactationを読んで、妊娠中および授乳中のアムロジ
ピンの使用について、以下の（　　　）内の空欄を埋めましょう。

Pregnancy（妊娠）

　　　　●ヒトの妊娠中におけるアムロジピンの安全性は（**1**　　　　　　　　　　　）。

　　　　●動物実験において、（**2**　　　　　　　　　　　　　　　）が観察された。

　　　　●妊娠中の使用は、（**3**　　　　　　　　　　　　　　　）推奨される。

Breast-feeding（授乳）

　　　　●アムロジピンが（**4**　　　　　　　　　　　　　　　）は不明である。

　　　　●授乳を継続/中止するか、あるいは、アムロジピンによる治療を継続/中止するかどうか
　　　　についての決断は、（**5**　　　　　　　　　　）を考慮に入れて判断されるべきである。

Exercise 3

A. 医療従事者向けのSmPCでは専門用語が多用されますが、患者や一般の人向けのPILでは平易
な表現が用いられます。副作用に関する表現について、下の表にあるSmPCに使用されている表
現とPILの表現（a～i）を対応させて、解答欄**1**～**9**を埋めましょう。

SmPCの表現

1 hyperglycaemia　(　　)	**4** aortic stenosis　　　　(　　)	**7** fatigue　　(　　)
2 hypotension　　(　　)	**5** impaired hepatic function　(　　)	**8** insomnia　(　　)
3 angina pectoris　(　　)	**6** nausea　　　　　　(　　)	**9** rhinitis　　(　　)

18 *Lesson 3*

PILの表現

a. tiredness	d. problems sleeping	g. raised blood sugar levels
b. narrowing of the heart valve of the aorta	e. liver disease	h. low blood pressure
c. feeling sick	f. sneezing/runny nose caused by inflammation of the lining of the nose	i. a certain type of chest pain

B. 次の文の**1**～**13**に入る前置詞を選択肢の中から選びましょう。音声を聞いて確認しましょう。

(🔊 Track03-1)

≪American English≫

1. Patients（**1** with / of / in）cardiac failure should be treated（**2** at / with / before）caution.

2. The safety and efficacy（**3** of / in / with）amlodipine（**4** by / in / of）hypertensive crisis has not been established.

3. Amlodipine should be initiated（**5** of / at / in）the lowest dose and titrated slowly（**6** by / of / in）patients with severe hepatic impairment.

4. Dosage recommendations have not been established（**7** up / in / by）patients with mild（**8** to / into / for）moderate hepatic impairment.

5. （**9** Up / For / On）both hypertension and angina, the usual initial dose is 5 mg amlodipine once daily which may be increased（**10** by / until / to）a maximum dose of 10 mg depending（**11** on / for / of）the individual patient's response.

6. （**12** From / In / By）hypertensive patients, amlodipine has been used in combination（**13** with / up / for）a thiazide diuretic, alpha blocker, beta blocker, or an angiotensin converting enzyme inhibitor.

19

Lesson 4

Media Literacy for Pharmacists
薬剤師のメディアリテラシー

　Lesson 2 では患者向け医薬品情報書PIL、Lesson 3 では医療従事者用添付文書SmPCを読んできましたが、Lesson 4 では、薬剤師が医薬品以外の情報を提供する場合の注意点とその情報の利用方法を取り上げます。

　インターネットは情報を探すのに大変便利ですが、検索サイトで目的の情報の関連語を検索するだけでは、ブログの記事やソーシャル・ネットワークの書き込みなど、医療従事者ではない人が書いた、根拠のない情報にたどり着いてしまう可能性もあります。薬剤師が情報提供をする際には、「根拠に基づく医療」(EBM: evidence based medicine)という言葉が表すように、信頼できる情報源から得たエビデンスに基づいた情報を利用しなければなりません。信頼できる情報源には、政府機関や学会、製薬企業などのウェブサイトなどがあげられます（pp. 24-25を参照）。

✏️▷ Getting to know the genre

Genre: 健康に関するアドバイス

● **Purpose:** 　　　　　　病気の予防方法を提案する

● **Audience:** 　　　　　　一般の人々

● **Information:** 　　　　　高血圧予防につながる生活習慣

● **Language features:**　専門知識を持たない人が理解できる平易な表現、見出し

🔍 Checking the terms

aim to	〜することを目標とする	portion	ポーション ※一盛り、などの意味だが、詳しくはEatwell Guide を参照。
artery	動脈		
cut down on	を減らす	pound	ポンド ※重量の単位。発音に注意
diet	食事、食事療法		
Eatwell Guide	イートウェル・ガイド* ※健康的な食事をするためにどの食物グループからどのぐらいの量を食べると良いのかを示した、イギリス政府によるガイドライン。	proportion	割合
		sleep deprivation	睡眠不足
		stroke	脳卒中
		surgery	診療所、医院、クリニック[英] ※手術[米]
fibre[英]	食物繊維		
heart attack	心臓発作	unit	ユニット ※ここでは酒の単位で、1ユニットは100％アルコールで10ml**
in moderation	適度に		
moderate-intensity aerobic activity	中強度の有酸素活動	6g of salt a day	1日に塩6グラム ※6 g は発音するときは "six grams" と複数形になる。
overweight	過体重		
plenty of	たくさんの〜		

*https://www.nhs.uk/live-well/eat-well/the-eatwell-guide/
**詳しくはPatient education: Alcohol use — when is drinking a problem? (Beyond the Basics)
https://www.uptodate.com/contents/alcohol-use-when-is-drinking-a-problem-beyond-the-basicsの "What is one drink?" を参照。

20　*Lesson 4*

Reading the text

Prevention: High blood pressure (hypertension)

https://www.nhs.uk/conditions/high-blood-pressure-hypertension/prevention/
Page last reviewed on May 21, 2019. Retrieved on July 22, 2019

High blood pressure can often be prevented or reduced by eating healthily, maintaining a healthy
weight, taking regular exercise, drinking alcohol in moderation and not smoking.

Healthy diet

Cut down on the amount of salt in your food and eat plenty of fruit and vegetables. The Eatwell
Guide highlights the different types of food that make up our diet, and shows the proportions we
should eat them in to have a well-balanced and healthy diet.

Salt raises your blood pressure. The more salt you eat, the higher your blood pressure. Aim to eat less
than 6 g (0.2 oz) of salt a day, which is about a teaspoonful.

Eating a low-fat diet that includes lots of fibre – such as wholegrain rice, bread and pasta – and plenty
of fruit and vegetables also helps lower blood pressure. Aim to eat five portions of fruit and vegetables
every day.

Limit your alcohol intake

Regularly drinking too much alcohol above recommended limits can raise your blood pressure over
time. Staying within these recommended levels is the best way to reduce your risk of developing
high blood pressure:

- men and women are advised not to regularly drink more than 14 units a week
- spread your drinking over three days or more if you drink as much as 14 units a week

Alcohol is also high in calories, which will make you gain weight and can further increase your
blood pressure.

Lose weight

Being overweight forces your heart to work harder to pump blood around your body, which can raise
your blood pressure. If you do need to lose some weight, it's worth remembering that just losing a
few pounds will make a big difference to your blood pressure and overall health.

Get active

Being active and taking regular exercise lowers blood pressure by keeping your heart and blood
vessels in good condition. Regular exercise can also help you lose weight, which will also help lower
your blood pressure. Adults should do at least 150 minutes (2 hours and 30 minutes) of moderate-
intensity aerobic activity such as cycling or fast walking every week. Physical activity can include
anything from sport to walking and gardening.

Cut down on caffeine

Drinking more than four cups of coffee a day may increase your blood pressure. If you're a big fan
of coffee, tea or other caffeine-rich drinks, such as cola and some energy drinks, consider cutting
down. It's fine to drink tea and coffee as part of a balanced diet, but it's important that these drinks
are not your main or only source of fluid.

Stop smoking

Smoking doesn't directly cause high blood pressure, but it puts you at much higher risk of a heart
attack and stroke. Smoking, like high blood pressure, will cause your arteries to narrow. If you
smoke and have high blood pressure, your arteries will narrow much more quickly, and your risk of
heart or lung disease in the future is dramatically increased.

Get a good night's sleep

Long-term sleep deprivation is associated with a rise in blood pressure and an increased risk of
hypertension. It's a good idea to try to get at least six hours of sleep a night.

Exercise 1

前ページの英文は、信頼できる医療情報源の1つ、イギリスの国営医療制度 National Health Service (NHS) のウェブサイト記事です。ここでは、皆さんが薬剤師として勤める薬局に外国人患者がやって来たという前提で、この記事を参照しながら情報提供の練習をしましょう。この患者は病院を受診した際に血圧が上昇傾向にあることを医師に指摘されたため、生活面での改善方法についてアドバイスを求めています。下線部に日本語で記されている薬剤師の会話の内容を前ページの Text を参考に英語に訳し、会話文を完成させましょう。

≪British English≫

Patient:　　　 Hello. Could you give me some advice? I was just told by the doctor at ABC Surgery that my blood pressure was getting a little high. Before taking any medications, he recommended me to try some life-style changes to lower the blood pressure. Could you tell me what I can do for that?

5　Pharmacist: Of course. First, you can 食事の塩分を減らす（**1**　　　　　　　　　　　　　　　　）.

Patient:　　　 OK. But why salt?

Pharmacist: Because 塩分を摂りすぎると、血圧が上がる（**2**　　　　　　　　　　　　　　）.

Patient:　　　 I see. I'll try. What else can I do?

Pharmacist: You can also アルコールの摂取量を制限する（**3**　　　　　　　　　　　　　）.

10　Patient:　　　 How much?

Pharmacist: 1週間に常習的に14ユニットを超えて飲まないようにと推奨されている

　　　　　　　（**4**　　　　　　　　　　　　　　　　　　　　　　　　　　　　　　）.

Patient:　　　 Hmm, what's a "unit"?

Pharmacist: A unit in this case refers to 10 ml of 100% alcohol. So you have to convert what you

15　　　　　　 drink into units. For example, six glasses of 13.5% wine roughly equals 14 units.

Patient:　　　 I think I usually drink less than that.

Pharmacist: That's good. 定期的に運動すること（**5**　　　　　　　　　　　　　） is also

　　　　　　 recommended.

　　　　　　 活動的でいて、定期的な運動をすると、心臓や血管を良い状態に保って血圧を下げる

20　　　　　　（**6**　　　　　　　　　　　　　　　　　　　　　　　　　　　　　　　　）.

Patient:　　　 Cut down on salt, limit alcohol intake, and regular exercise. I think I got it. Thank you.

　　会話が完成したら、音声を聞いて答え合わせをしましょう。　　　　　　　　　（ •))| **Track04-1**）
　　次に、薬剤師役と外国人患者役に分かれて会話の練習をしましょう。

Exercise 2

英語では、動名詞（動詞原形に ing をつけた形で、動詞を名詞化したもの）を利用して主語にすることができます。1. から 4. までの下線部の動詞を適切な形に変えて文法的に正しい文にしましょう。次に、文の主語（主部）と動詞（述部）がどこかを書き出し、文全体の意味を考えましょう。

22　*Lesson 4*

1. Regularly <u>drink</u> alcohol above recommended limits can raise your blood pressure over time.

　　主語（主部）：**1**

　　動詞（述部）：**2**

　　訳：**3**

2. <u>Be</u> overweight forces your heart to work harder to pump blood around your body.

　　主語（主部）：**4**

　　動詞（述部）：**5**

　　訳：**6**

3. <u>Be</u> active and <u>take</u> regular exercise lowers blood pressure by keeping your heart and blood vessels in good condition.

　　主語（主部）：**7**

　　動詞（述部）：**8**

　　訳：**9**

4. <u>Drink</u> more than four cups of coffee a day may increase your blood pressure.

　　主語（主部）：**10**

　　動詞（述部）：**11**

　　訳：**12**

✏➤ Exercise 3

生活習慣の改善法をアドバイスする以下の文を、Reading the text を参考に英語で表現しましょう。

1 1日に摂取する塩分量を小さじ1杯程度、6 g未満にすることを目標にしましょう。

2 もし週に14ユニット程度飲酒するようであれば、3日以上に分けるようにしましょう。

3 数キログラム体重を減らすだけでも、血圧や健康に大きなメリットがあるということを覚えておくと良いでしょう。

4 バランスの取れた食事の一部として紅茶やコーヒーを飲むのは大丈夫ですが、これらがあなたの水分補給の主要な、もしくは唯一の飲料とならないように気をつけなければなりません。

5 1晩に少なくとも6時間は眠るようにすると良いでしょう。

23

Applying what you learned

薬局に勤める薬剤師として、高血圧の治療をしている外国人患者に以下の点についてアドバイスしましょう。**1**～**6**のうち興味のあるものを選び、UpToDateの患者向けウェブサイト（https://www.uptodate.com/patients/）にアクセスして、必要な情報を調べましょう（UpToDateについての説明は下記参照）。一度検索しただけでは回答の得られる最適なウェブページにたどり着けないかもしれませんので、関連ページの中のリンクもたどってみましょう。

1 減塩する時、何に気を付ければ良いか？

2 お酒（ビール1, 2缶またはグラスワイン1杯約150 ml／回）を週4回程度飲むのは適量か？

3 どうして魚を食べることが体に良いのか教えてほしい。

4 食物繊維を取りたいが、何を食べると良いか？

5 コーヒーは血圧にどのような影響を与えるか？　1日に何杯くらいまでが適当か？

6 The DASH Eating Planについて説明してもらいたい。

医療情報を収集するための信頼のおける情報源の一例を以下に紹介します。調べものをする際に、ぜひ活用してみてください。

UpToDate https://www.uptodate.com/

　UpToDateは日本を含め世界中の医療機関で信頼できる情報源として利用されているウェブサイトです。ここにはエビデンスに基づいた最新の情報が寄せられており、治療方針を決定する際の参考にも利用されます。また医療従事者向けの情報だけでなく、患者の教育のための情報も提供されています。日本の病院の薬剤部ではDI（Drug Information）活動に欠かせない情報源の1つといえます。病院や薬局等では有料ユーザーとして登録していることが多いですが、上のApplying what you learnedでは誰でも利用できる患者向けページを使っています。

イギリス国民保健サービス　National Health Service（NHS）

https://www.nhs.uk/

　イギリスの国営医療制度。Health A-Zコーナーでは病気の症状、治療法についてや、症状が出ている時に何をすべきか、いつ病院に行くべきか等の情報を、Medicine A-Zコーナーでは薬の効果、飲み方、副作用などの情報を提供しています。

24 *Lesson 4*

アメリカ食品医薬品局　U.S. Food and Drug Administration（FDA）

https://www.fda.gov/

　アメリカ保健社会福祉省の下部機関で、食品、食品添加物、タバコ、医薬品、玩具、医療機器などの製品の品質、衛生管理、宣伝などについて規制を行っています。ウェブサイトには上記分野を含む幅広い情報が掲載されており、またFor Consumer, Patients, Health Professionals, Industryなど利用者に合わせた情報を見ることもできます。

アメリカ疾病管理予防センター　Centers for Disease Control and Prevention（CDC）

https://www.cdc.gov/

　アメリカ保健社会福祉省の下部機関で、感染症対策の研究を行い、また健康に関する種々の決定の根拠となる信頼できる情報の提供を行っています。ウェブサイトには感染症の発生に対応する方法などはもちろん、一般的な疾病についての情報、健康的な生活を送るためのコツ、旅行者が旅先で気をつけるべきことなどの情報も提供されています。

アメリカ国立衛生研究所　National Institutes of Health（NIH）　https://www.nih.gov/

　アメリカ保健社会福祉省の下部機関で、がん、老化、アルコール依存症、アレルギーなどの様々な研究を行う施設が集まっています。ウェブサイトではそのような施設での研究の最新情報に加え、非医療従事者向けに簡単な言葉で書かれた健康情報なども提供されています。

メイヨー・クリニック　Mayo Clinic　https://www.mayoclinic.org/

　アメリカ合衆国ミネソタ州にある総合病院で、アメリカ合衆国の中で最も優れた病院の一つと考えられています。ウェブサイトでは通常の病院業務に関する情報（予約を取る、所属医師を探す等）の他、症状を選んでいくとその原因だと考えられる病気を提案するSymptom Checkerなどもあります。

MSD Manuals　https://www.msdmanuals.com/

　アメリカ合衆国に本社を置くメルク・アンド・カンパニー社が運営する医学マニュアルで、米国ではMerck Manual、その他の国ではMSDマニュアルという名称で知られています。すべての人が正確かつ役立つ医学情報にアクセスする権利をもっているという信念に基づき、膨大な、信頼のおける情報を英語だけでなく、ポルトガル語、中国語、日本語など多言語で無償提供しています。

MedlinePlus　https://medlineplus.gov/

　アメリカ国立衛生研究所の一部門で、世界最大の医学図書館であるアメリカ国立医学図書館のウェブサイト。健康、薬、サプリメントについての情報に加え、健康に関する英語字幕付き動画や健康状態をチェックするリスト等も豊富に用意されています。

Lesson *5*

FDA Website Information on Clinical Trials
臨床試験に関するFDAのウェブサイト情報

　Clinical Trial（臨床試験、治験）とは、医薬品の安全性と有効性について詳しく調べるために行うヒトを対象とした研究です。各国の規制当局は、医薬品の研究開発過程から得られた膨大な情報を審査し、その結果承認された医薬品だけが販売を許可されて患者のもとに届けられます。医薬品が市販されると、さまざまな年齢層、人種（race）、民族（ethnicity）の人々が使用する可能性があります。そのため、治験にはできるだけ幅広い参加者を組み入れることが望まれます。

　Lesson 5では、米国の食品医薬品局（Food and Drug Administration: FDA）が掲載したウェブサイト記事を紹介します。多民族国家の米国で少数派の人々（minority）が治験に参加することの重要性についてどのように述べられているか学びましょう。

Getting to know the genre

Genre: 政府機関が掲載したウェブサイト上の記事

- **Purpose:** 　　　　　　医療に関する情報を一般の人にわかりやすく説明する
- **Audience:** 　　　　　　医療専門家でない一般の人々
- **Information:** 　　　　　問題点の指摘と展望
- **Language features:** 非専門用語の使用、読みやすくするための見出し

Checking the terms

agency	機関、当局 ※ここではFDAをさす		**oversight**	監視
			patient advocate	患者擁護者
antidepressant	抗うつ薬		**proactive**	積極的な、前向きな
application	（新薬などの承認）申請		**public health**	公衆衛生
disparity	不均衡		**regulatory**	規制の
disproportionately	不釣り合いに、偏って		**represent**	（ある集団を）代表する
diversity	多様性		**subject**	臨床試験の被験者
effectiveness	有効性		**syphilis**	梅毒
genetic coding	遺伝暗号（化）		**undergo**	（治療や検査を）受ける
lay people	専門知識を持たない一般人		**under-represented**	十分に代表していない
marketing approval	販売承認		**vulnerable**	脆弱な

Reading the text

Clinical Trials Shed Light on Minority Health

https://wayback.archive-it.org/7993/20171101162929/https://www.fda.gov/ForConsumers/ConsumerUpdates/ucm349063.htm

The Food and Drug Administration (FDA) is working to increase the participation of people in racial, ethnic and other minority groups in the clinical trials that test new medical products.

5 Why is this important?
Ensuring meaningful representation of minorities in clinical trials for regulated medical products is fundamental to FDA's regulatory mission and public health, says Jonca Bull, M.D., director of the agency's Office of Minority Health (OMH). Racial and ethnic minorities include African American, American Indian, Alaska Native, Asian American, Hispanic American, Native Hawaiian and Pacific
10 Islander communities.
OMH project manager Christine Merenda, M.P.H., R.N. explains that clinical trials are the proving ground for new drugs, vaccines and devices. They provide the data that will determine whether FDA approves a manufacturer's application for marketing approval.
"Potential racial, ethnic and other differences in response to drugs are important to FDA's efforts to
15 help ensure that the safety and effectiveness of drugs are studied in all people who will use the products once they are approved," she says.

Considering Genetic Differences
Bull explains that there are biological differences in how people process drugs. For example, (1) variations in genetic coding can make a cancer treatment more toxic in one ethnic group than it
20 would be in another. These variations can also make drugs like antidepressants and blood-pressure medications less effective in one group than another.
Getting more data on these differences is essential for FDA to truly know that a medical product will truly work and be safe for all patients, Bull says.

Members of minority groups may be more vulnerable to certain diseases. "We know, for example,
25 that (2) African-Americans and Hispanics have higher rates of diabetes, HIV/AIDS, obesity and cardiovascular disease," says Bull. Native Americans and Asians have been shown to have higher rates of hepatitis, while Hispanics are disproportionately affected by diabetes.

But historically, both women and minorities have been under-represented in clinical trials. For example, according to a 2011 report from the conference "Dialogues on Diversifying Clinical
30 Trials," sponsored by FDA's Office of Women' s Health and the Society for Women's Health Research and supported by OMH:
● African Americans represent 12% of the U.S. population but only 5% of clinical trial participants;
● Hispanics make up 16% of the population but only 1% of clinical trial participants; and
● Men make up more than two-thirds of the participants in clinical tests of cardiovascular (heart and
35 blood vessel) devices.
At the conference, more than 200 representatives from government and industry came together with patient advocates and the scientific community to discuss strategies for increasing the participation of women and minorities in clinical trials.

Why the Disparity?

40 Bull says there are different reasons why minorities have been under-represented in clinical trials. (3) One reason may be a lack of trust because of past abuses, Bull says. One notorious example was the Tuskegee Syphilis Study, experiments conducted between 1932 and 1972 by the U.S. Public Health Service. Health officials recruited poor black sharecroppers in Alabama to study the natural progress of syphilis. However, while the study was in progress, penicillin was discovered to treat

45 syphilis. The study was not stopped and the men were not treated with penicillin that could have cured them.

According to a recent university study, however, this attitude seems to be changing. (4) The study was designed to learn the health concerns and research perceptions among under-represented groups. When asked about their overall interest in medical research, 91 percent of African-Americans

50 expressed interest in participating.

Nonetheless, recruiting people to participate in clinical trials—no matter what race or ethnicity—is difficult in general, Bull notes. FDA works to protect participants in clinical trials and to ensure that people have reliable information as they decide whether to join a clinical trial.

There are many benefits to minority participation for researchers that extend, in a larger sense, to

55 society. Minority participation helps researchers find better treatments and better ways to fight such diseases as cancer, diabetes, heart disease and HIV/AIDS. In addition, it uncovers differences by gender, race, and ethnicity that may be important for safe and effective use of therapies.

Safeguards and Resources

(5) Safeguards for clinical trial participants include oversight by institutional review boards (IRBs),

60 composed of at least five members, including scientists, doctors, and lay people. IRBs ensure that appropriate steps are taken to protect the rights and welfare of participants as subjects of research. Though it's too soon to tell, Bull says that the FDA Safety and Innovation Act (FDASIA) signed into law by President Obama in July 2012 could have a helpful effect in supporting efforts to enhance minority participation in clinical trials. FDASIA requires that FDA report to Congress by July 9,

65 2013 on the diversity of participants in clinical trials and the extent to which safety and effectiveness data based on such factors as sex, age, race and ethnicity are included in applications submitted to FDA.

Based on these findings, FDA and others involved in clinical research will be able to identify needs and opportunities to increase minority representation, says Bull.

70 In the meantime, Bull encourages consumers to take a more proactive approach. (6) If you're undergoing treatment and your condition is not improving, she says, you may want to talk to your health care professional about the availability of clinical trials that address your condition.

April 26, 2013

※FDA archive について

この記事は現在アーカイブ化（保管文書化）されています。日進月歩の医学分野では情報が常に更新され、古い記事は順次アーカイブ化されます。過去のFDA記事は、FDAウェブサイトからアーカイブページ（FDA.gov Archive）に入り、記事のタイトルで検索することができます。アーカイブ化された記事は、アップロードされた時点でのURLではアクセスできなくなることに注意しましょう。

Exercise 1

A. 本文中に記載されている人種・民族的に少数派の人々（racial and ethnic minorities）を表す表現について、次の表に整理しましょう。また、Exercise 2 に race, ethnicity, minority についてのより詳細な問題がありますので確認しておきましょう。

Racial and ethnic minorities	日本語
African American	**1**
American Indian	**2**
Alaska Native	**3**
Asian American	**4**
Hispanic American	**5**
Native Hawaiian	**6**
Pacific Islander	**7**

B. 薬に対する反応は、人種や民族の違いに起因する生物学的差異によって異なる可能性があると説明されています。具体的にどのような薬で何が起こる可能性があるのか、本文の下線部 (1) の内容を日本語で説明しましょう。

1

C. 人種・民族的に少数派の人々が他の民族よりも有病率が高い病気についても紹介されています。本文の下線部 (2) の内容を以下の表にまとめましょう。

Racial and ethnic minorities	他の民族よりも有病率が高い病気
African-Americans and Hispanics	**1**
Native Americans and Asians	**2**

D. 人種・民族的に少数派の人々は、薬に対する反応や病気に対する脆弱性が異なる可能性がある一方、臨床試験でこれら少数派の人々および女性は人口比にみあった数の人々が参加していない（under-represented）と説明されています。本文中の 3 つの箇条書きを次の表にまとめましょう。

29

	全人口に占める割合	治験参加者に占める割合
African-Americans	**1**	**3**
Hispanics	**2**	**4**
Men*	$\dfrac{1}{2}$	**5**

*心血管系で使用する医療機器の臨床試験への参加者

E. 臨床試験への少数派の人々の参加割合が不均衡である理由の一つとして、Tuskegee Syphilis Studyの出来事が紹介されています。本文の下線部(3)の部分の内容を日本語で説明しましょう。

※ Tuskegee Syphilis Studyの詳細は、Center for Disease Control and Prevention（CDC: 米国疾病対策センター）の以下のウェブサイトに記述されています。https://www.cdc.gov/tuskegee/timeline.htm

1

F. ある大学の研究結果によると状況は改善してきているようです。本文の下線部(4)に示されているこの研究の内容を説明しましょう。

この研究の目的	**1**
結果	**2**

G. FDAや厚生労働省など各国の薬事当局は、臨床試験の参加者を保護するため、環境を整備しています。その手段の一つとして、この記事にはInstitutional Review Board (IRB)による監視が紹介されています。IRBはEthics Committee（倫理委員会）と呼ばれることもあり、臨床試験を実施する医療機関に設置することが義務付けられている委員会です。IRBに関する本文の下線部(5)の記述内容を次の表にまとめましょう。

Institutional Review Board (IRB)	日本語:**1**
IRBの構成員	日本語:**2**
IRBの目的	日本語:**3**

30 *Lesson 5*

※日本製薬工業協会（製薬協、Japan Pharmaceutical Manufacturers Association：JPMA）が一般の人々を対象に治験について紹介している以下のウェブサイトも参考にしてください。

製薬協「治験について」：http://www.jpma.or.jp/medicine/shinyaku/tiken/tiken/

H. 記事の最後には、人々が治験への参加により積極的なアプローチをとることを推奨するという記述があります。本文の下線部(6)の内容から、その理由を考察してみましょう。

> **1**

患者が薬剤師に治験について相談することも少なくありません。治験に関する情報は、この記事で紹介されているNational Institute of Health（NIH: 米国国立衛生研究所）のClinicalTrials. govで全世界の治験や臨床研究情報が検索できるほか、日本にも以下のウェブサイトがあります。

・臨床試験情報（一般財団法人　日本医薬情報センター）：https://www.clinicaltrials.jp
・臨床研究情報ポータルサイト（国立保健医療科学院）：https://rctportal.niph.go.jp/

✏️ Exercise 2

臨床試験における人種・民族の取り扱いについてはFDA Guidance*に規定されており、人種(race)については以下の説明**があります。また、音声を聞き、人種や国の名称の正しい発音を練習しましょう。

*Collection of Race and Ethnicity Data in Clinical Trials Guidance for Industry and Food and Drug Administration Staff
 https://www.fda.gov/media/75453/download
**一部省略

American Indian or Alaska Native: A person having origins in any of the original peoples of North and South America (including Central America), and who maintains tribal affiliation or community attachment.

Asian: A person having origins in any of the original peoples of the Far East, Southeast Asia, or the Indian subcontinent, including, for example, Cambodia, China, India, Japan, Korea, Malaysia, Pakistan, the Philippine Islands, Thailand, and Vietnam.

Black or African American: A person having origins in any of the black racial groups of Africa.

Native Hawaiian or Other Pacific Islander: A person having origins in any of the original peoples of Hawaii, Guam, Samoa, or other Pacific Islands.

White: A person having origins in any of the original peoples of Europe, the Middle East, or North Africa.

A. FDA Guidanceに記載されているそれぞれの人種にはどの地域を起源とする人が含まれるのか、下のボックスにある選択肢を表に当てはめましょう。

(🔊 Track05-1)

White	Black or African American	American Indian or Alaska Native	Asian	Native Hawaiian or Other Pacific Islander
1	**2**	**3**	**4**	**5**

インド亜大陸	北アフリカ	北アメリカ	極東	グアム	サモア諸島
太平洋諸島	中東	中央アメリカ	東南アジア	ハワイ	南アメリカ
ヨーロッパ	アフリカ				

民族 (ethnicity)については以下の説明があります。

For ethnicity, we recommend the following minimum choices be offered:

Hispanic or Latino: A person of Cuban, Mexican, Puerto Rican, South or Central American, or other Spanish culture or origin, regardless of race. The term, "Spanish origin," can be used in addition to "Hispanic or Latino."

Not Hispanic or Latino

B. 上記の**Hispanic or Latino**の説明を日本語に訳しましょう。

米国国勢調査局による説明***では、race (人種) とethnicity(民族)は二つの異なる独立した概念として以下のように定義されています。

***US Census Bureau "Race and Ethnicity": https://www.census.gov/mso/www/training/pdf/race-ethnicity-onepager.pdf#search='race+ethnicity+difference

What is race?

The Census Bureau defines race as a person's self-identification with one or more social groups.

32 *Lesson 5*

An individual can report as White, Black or African American, Asian, American Indian and Alaska Native, Native Hawaiian and Other Pacific Islander, or some other race. Survey respondents may report multiple races.

What is ethnicity?

Ethnicity determines whether a person is of Hispanic origin or not. For this reason, ethnicity is broken out in two categories, Hispanic or Latino and Not Hispanic or Latino. Hispanics may report as any race.

C. 上記の説明をもとに、race(人種)とethnicity(民族)は概念としてどのように異なるのか、グループで話し合いましょう。また音声も聞きましょう。 (⁍ Track05-2)

⟹ Applying what you learned

医薬品の研究開発（Research and Development: R&D）に関する以下の事柄について、FDAやその他のウェブサイトを参照しながらグループで内容をまとめて発表しましょう。

■ 医薬品の研究開発過程はどのようになっているか？

■ 前臨床試験はどのような基準に基づいて実施されるか？

■ 臨床試験の4つのフェーズとは何か？

■ インフォームドコンセントとは何か？どのような情報を含める必要があるか？

■ FDAの医薬品審査過程はどのようになっているか？

■ FDAの市販後の医薬品モニタリングはどのようになっているか？

※日本の薬事当局である厚生労働省でも、一般の人を対象とした治験に関するウェブサイトが用意されています。また、日本における医薬品と医療機器の承認審査や市販後の安全性情報収集については、独立行政法人 医薬品医療機器総合機構（Pharmaceuticals and Medical Devices Agency：Pmda）のウェブサイトに詳細が記載されています。

治験について（一般向け）：https://www.mhlw.go.jp/stf/seisakunitsuite/bunya/fukyu.html
医薬品医療機器総合機構（Pmda）：http://www.pmda.go.jp/index.html

Lesson 6

Medication Counseling 1
服薬指導(1)　初回面談・薬歴記載

　日本には多くの在留外国人がいます。自国で処方された薬をもって来日していても、医薬品医療機器等法により日本に持ち込める薬の量に制限があります*ので、いずれ日本で処方を受けなくてはならなくなります。Lesson 6では、処方箋をもって初来局した外国人患者との面談や服薬指導、薬歴の記載、求められた情報を提供するために情報収集をして英語で情報提供します。

*https://www.mhlw.go.jp/english/policy/health-medical/pharmaceuticals/01.html（厚生労働省ホームページ）
　http://www.customs.go.jp/tetsuzuki/c-answer/imtsukan/1806_jr.htm（税関ホームページ）

Getting to know the genre

Genre：初回面談・服薬指導の会話

● **Purpose**:　　　　　安全に薬を提供するため、初来局の患者から情報を聞き取り、服薬指導する

● **Audience***:　　　　薬剤師・初来局の外国人患者（とその家族）

● **Information**:　　　　患者の病歴や体質などの情報、投薬する薬の情報

● **Language features**:　専門知識を持たない人が理解できる平易な表現、見出し

*ここでは participants「本書の内容構成と使い方」参照

Checking the terms

antihypertensive drug	抗高血圧薬	health insurance	健康保険
asthma	喘息	hypoglycemia[*]	低血糖症
bear with me	もう少し待ってください	irritating	チカチカ、イガイガする
(food) being off	（食べ物が）悪くなっている	itchy	痒い
clinic	（主に米）診療所、医院	mackerel	鯖
combination tablet	複数の成分を含む配合錠	moderately	程々に
complication	合併症	out-of-pocket	自己負担で
counseling[*]	カウンセリング	physician	医師、内科医
develop	（病気を）発症する	rash	発疹
dispense	調剤する	religion	宗教
enlarged prostate	前立腺肥大症	social drinker	付き合い程度に飲酒する人
(100)°F (Fahrenheit)	華氏(100)度（= 37.8℃）	thyroid disease	甲状腺の病気
		tingling sensation	ヒリヒリ、チクチクする感覚
HbA1c (hemoglobin A1c)	グリコヘモグロビン	tremor	震え

34　*Lesson 6*

Reading the text

処方箋を持って初来局した外国人患者との初回面談

調剤薬局に初来局した患者には、処方された薬が併用薬やサプリメントと相互作用がないか、生活習慣によって副作用が増強される可能性がないか質問します。次の会話文の音声を聞きましょう。

（◀ｻ **Track06-1**）

≪American English≫

Pharmacist:	Good afternoon, Mrs. Victoria. (1) <u>I'm Nozomi Yamamoto,</u> <u>your pharmacist.</u> Because this is your first visit to this pharmacy, may I ask you some questions?
Patient:	Oh, yes. Of course.
5 Pharmacist:	(2) <u>Do you have health insurance?</u>
Patient:	Yes, I have *Kenko Hoken*. This is my *Kenko Hoken* card.
Pharmacist:	Oh, good. Is this the first time you have visited a physician in Japan using *Kenko Hoken*?
Patient:	Yes, it's the first time. I know I have to pay 30% of the total
10	cost for medication. Do you accept a credit card?
Pharmacist:	You have to pay 30% out-of-pocket. I'm afraid we only accept cash.
Patient:	Ok. I guess it won't be so expensive.
Pharmacist:	(3) <u>To make sure the medicines we dispense are appropriate</u>
15	<u>and safe for you to take, let me ask you some questions about</u> <u>your physical and medical background.</u>
Patient:	That's fine, please go ahead.
Pharmacist:	Are you taking any other medication?
Patient:	Not regularly.
20 Pharmacist:	Have you taken any over the counter drug for the current problem?
Patient:	Oh, I took Tylenol last night, which I brought from the US, as my temperature was high.
Pharmacist:	How high was it? (4) <u>Do you remember the dosage?</u>
25 Patient:	It was 100° F. I took two tablets. I think it's 500 mg per tablet.
Pharmacist:	Thank you. Do you have any allergy to any medicine or food?
Patient:	No, I don't think so.
Pharmacist:	(5) <u>Have you ever been unwell after eating a particular food?</u>
Patient:	Ah, yes. I sometimes feel a tingling sensation in my throat
30	when I eat kiwi fruit. And on one occasion, I had an irritating and itchy rash after eating mackerel but I think the mackerel was a bit off.
Pharmacist:	I see. (6) <u>Is there anything you cannot consume due to your</u> <u>religion?</u>
35 Patient:	No, nothing like that.

下線部分のポイント：

(1) 自己紹介。名札に薬剤師と書いてあっても外国人にはわからないこともある。

(2) 保険の確認は必要。長期滞在者は日本の健康保険を持っていることが基本だが、旅行者は保険を持っていなかったり、旅行傷害保険を使って医療機関を受診したりすることがある。

(3) 初回面談を行う必要性を述べる。

(4) 服用中の薬やサプリメントの量も重要な情報。

(5) 1つ前の質問でアレルギーについて聞いているが、アレルギーの定義は一般人にはわかりにくいので、言葉を変えて聞く。

(6) たとえばイスラム教徒やヒンズー教徒には豚や牛由来の成分の入った薬は提供できないことがある（例：牛豚由来の消化酵素が含まれた消化剤）。

35

Pharmacist: Do you drink alcohol?

Patient: I only drink moderately at parties. I'm a social drinker.

Exercise 1

A. 初回面談の会話で利用できる表現を考えましょう。1. から5. の英文の空欄に入る適当な表現を入れましょう。空欄に適した単語は1つとは限りません。文法上問題がない単語を入れましょう。6. から10. は日本語を英語に訳しましょう。音声を聞いて答え合わせをしましょう。

(◀) Track 06-2)

※特に、動詞の時制を意識して考えましょう。
・現在形：好き嫌いなどの事実や習慣的に行なっていること（例：喫煙、飲酒、車の運転、運動）
・現在進行形：現時点で継続中のこと（例：現在服用中の薬剤やサプリメント）
・現在完了形：これまでの病歴、入院歴、アレルギーなど
・過去形：過去の一時点で起こったこと（去年入院した、一昨年手術したなど）

1. Are you currently (**1**   ) any medicines?
2. Have you ever (**2**   ) itchiness, rash, difficulty in breathing after
   (**3**   ) any food or (**4**   ) any medicine? If so, what are they?
3. Do you (**5**   ) any supplements or herbal medicines?
4. How many (**6**   ) of beer do you (**7**   ) a day?
5. When (**8**   ) stop smoking?
6. 普段、運動をしますか？　(**9**   )
7. 妊娠の可能性はありますか？　(**10**   )
8. タバコを吸いますか？一日にどの位吸いますか？　(**11**   )
9. これまでに重い病気にかかったことはありますか？　(**12**   )
10. これまでに入院されたことはありますか？　(**13**   )

B. 次ページは初回面談で使う英語の質問票例です。このLessonの会話を参考にして、この内容について薬剤師が患者に確認する会話の練習をしてみましょう。できるだけ情報を得るため、質問はYes-Noで答えるものだけではなく、Wh-疑問文、患者の答えに対する追加質問など工夫をしましょう。モデル会話の音声も聞きましょう。

(◀) Track 06-3)

① 各自、架空の患者としてすべての項目に回答する（自分自身のことでなくてよい）。
② ペアになって完成した質問票を交換し、相手の質問票を見て内容を確認する。
③ 薬剤師役と患者役となって、質問票の確認をするロールプレイを行う。

36　*Lesson 6*

Medical Questionnaire

Medical history is important for your safe medication use. Please answer the following questions. All information provided will be kept confidential.

Name: _____ DOB*: _____ Age:_____ y.o.**

Height: _____(cm/feet) Weight: _____(kg/lb) Body temperature: _____(°C/°F)

- Allergies:
  - □No □Yes → (_____)

- Current medications:
  - □No □Yes → (_____)
    - Names and dosage of the medications

- Supplements:
  - □No □Yes → (_____)
    - Names and dosage of the supplements

- Medical history:
  - If yes, circle the name of the disease(s).
  - High blood pressure   Diabetes   Heart disease
  - Liver disease   Dyslipidemia   Asthma
  - Thyroid disease   Enlarged prostate Glaucoma
  - Other (_____)

- Smoking:
  - □No □Rarely □Yes_____cigarettes/a day □Quit since age _____

- Drinking:
  - □No □Rarely □Yes_____times/a week;
    - Amount per day (   )

- Check the following if applicable:
  - □I drive a car or motorcycle.   □I operate dangerous machinery.
  - □I work in elevated places (for example, using a boom lift, working on scaffolding).

For women:
- Pregnancy:
  - □No □Yes:_____months pregnant □I don't know

- Breast-feeding: □No □Yes

Thank you for your cooperation.

This questionnaire will be used only for your treatment and not for other purposes.

*Date of Birthの略
**years oldの略

➡️ Exercise 2

SOAP形式の薬歴について

調剤薬局では、患者への調剤・投薬履歴となる薬歴を作成します。薬歴には、どの薬がいつ何日分処方されたか、投薬時にどのような聞き取りや指導を行ったか、などの情報が記されます。この際、S (subjective) O (objective) A (assessment) P (plan)の4つに分けて記します。基本的には、Sには「患者の言ったこと」、Oには「薬剤師から見た客観的事実、検査値など」、Aには「薬剤師の判断や行動」、Pには「計画」が記されます。書き方にはいろいろなスタイルがあります。特にSは、患者の言ったこと、心配している内容などのポイントを要約する書き方もありますが、患者の話した通りに書く場合もあります。外国人の場合は、どのような表現を患者が用いたか、どのような表現で薬剤師が説明したかがその後の服薬指導等で重要になることもありますから、Exercise 2では「患者が言ったこと」「患者に言ったこと」についてはどのような英語表現を使ったか記載しましょう。

A. 処方箋を持って、50代イギリス人男性のRichard Bickleyさんがあなたの薬局にやってきました。処方内容は、次の通りです。会話文をよく読んで、空欄 **1**〜**10** に入る単語を下のリストから選んで埋めましょう。次に、音声を聞いて **1**〜**10** の答え合わせをし、空欄 **11**〜**20** に入る言葉を聞き取って書き入れましょう。　　　　　　　　（ ◀))) **Track 06-4**）

処方	変更不可	個々の処方薬について、後発医薬品（ジェネリック医薬品）への変更に差し支えがあると判断した場合には、「変更不可」欄に「✓」又は「×」を記載し、「保険医署名」欄に署名又は記名・押印すること。 【般】シタグリプチン 50 mg錠　1錠　　　x 14日分 分1 朝食後 以下余白

breakfast	eaten	lab	less	reduce
develop	healthy	last	may	taken

≪British English≫

Pharmacist: Hello.

Patient: Hi. I visited a clinic today and got this prescription and I have some questions.

Pharmacist: How (**1**　　) I help you, Mr Bickley?

Patient: My doctor told me that my blood sugar is a bit high and he prescribed something to (**2**　　) the sugar level. What is this? He didn't tell me much, but how bad is my blood sugar?

Pharmacist: May I have a look at your (**3**　　) data? Hmmm, did you have (**4**　　) before your blood was (**5**　　)?

38　*Lesson 6*

| Patient: | No, I didn't. I still haven't (**6**   ) anything, so I am starving! |

10 Pharmacist: Your fasting blood sugar this morning was 180 mg/dL and HbA1c was 7.2%. Both are quite high and fall into the criteria for diabetes. The blood sugar level of (**7**   ) people at fasting is (**8**   ) than 100 mg/dL and the HbA1c is 5.5% or lower.

Patient: Hmmm. Oh, my numbers are really high. What is HbA1c? And why is high HbA1c bad?

15 Pharmacist: HbA1c reflects your blood sugar level for the (**9**   ) one to two months. If you have high HbA1c, you are more likely to (**10**   ) diabetes complications.

Patient: Hmmm, I've heard about diabetes complications like going blind or losing feet.

Pharmacist: Well, that's the worst case scenario. To reduce the risk for developing such complications, you have been prescribed a new medicine called sitagliptin. Take one tablet every

20 morning after breakfast. There is a possibility of lowering the blood sugar too much and you may experience hypoglycaemia. Symptoms of hypoglycaemia are feeling (**11**   ), (**12**   ), sick, (**13**   ), or (**14**   ), and tremors. If you feel such (**15**   ), eat some sweets or drink (**16**   ) like cola. Make sure the sweets or drink contain sugar but not (**17**   ) sweetener. When

25 you have a (**18**   ), (**19**   ) or (**20**   ), your blood sugar level may become unstable. So, please look after yourself more when you are ill.

Patient: Hmmm, sounds scary, but I will take this medicine.

Pharmacist: Good! Bear with me a moment. Let me check before you go. Could you tell me what this medicine is for? When to take it and how many tablets?

30 Patient: It's to reduce my blood sugar level. I should take one tablet after breakfast.

Pharmacist: What should you be careful about and what should you do if it happens?

Patient: I should be careful about low blood sugar. If it happens, I should have some sweets or sugar-containing drink.

Pharmacist: Perfect! If you have any concerns after taking this medicine, please do not hesitate to

35 contact us, Mr Bickley.

Patient: Thank you. I'm going to have breakfast soon and take the first one. Bye!

Pharmacist: Thank you. Take care.

B. 上の服薬指導を終えて、SOAP形式で薬歴を書いてみましょう。SやAで患者や薬剤師が実際に使ったキーワードは、英語の表現も含めて薬歴に残すようにしましょう。

S: (**1**   )

O:(**2**   )

A: 高血糖値を指摘され、シタグリプチン初処方。高血糖のリスクと血糖降下剤による低血糖症状とその対処法について次のように説明した。(**3**   )

P: 体調の変化がなかったか、低血糖症状の有無聞き取り。

Exercise 3

Valerie Alexandra さんは30代の米国から来日したアフリカ系アメリカ人の女性科学者です。彼女はテルミサルタン80 mg/ヒドロクロロチアジド12.5 mgの配合錠で2年間高血圧の治療を受けてきましたが、最近血圧コントロールが不良な状態が続いています。そのため、今回薬が変更になり、右のような処方箋をもって来局しました。次の流れに沿って薬剤師と患者の会話を作りましょう。

A. 薬剤師から患者へ伝えること
今回アムロジピンが追加処方されましたが、1錠追加されたのではなく、これまでの2種類の降圧薬の配合錠にアムロジピンが加わった3種類の配合錠が処方されていることを説明します。以下の会話文の音声を聞き、音読しましょう。(◀)) **Track 06-5**)

≪American English≫

Pharmacist: Ms. Alexandra, your doctor changed your medicine. Did he tell you about it?

Patient: Yes, he did. He said that he would add one more antihypertensive drug.

Pharmacist: How was your blood pressure today at the clinic?

Patient: It was 150/88 mmHg. I have been taking the medication properly, but it is still high.

5 Pharmacist: I see why he added a new medicine. Your blood pressure has been around 150/90 mmHg for the past few weeks, hasn't it? The new medicine is called amlodipine and it is a calcium channel blocker. You have been taking a telmisartan and hydrochlorothiazide combination tablet. You are not going to take one extra tablet, as there is a combination tablet of telmisartan, hydrochlorothiazide, and amlodipine.

10 Patient: Oh, that's good. I don't want to take too many tablets.

40 *Lesson 6*

B. グレープフルーツジュースとの相互作用について説明します。

1.アムロジピン服用中はグレープフルーツを摂取できないことを説明する会話文を、次の**1**～**12**に入る適切な言葉を考えて完成させましょう。音声を聞き、答え合わせをしましょう。　　　（ 🔊 **Track06-6**）

Pharmacist: (**1**　　　　　　　　　) you are (**2**　　　　　　　　　　　) amlodipine, please do not
(**3**　　　　　　　　) grapefruit juice or (**4**　　　　　　　　　　) grapefruit.

Patient: Really? So, I (**5**　　　　　　　　　) not (**6**　　　　　　　　) grapefruit in any
form.

5　Pharmacist: No, you (**7**　　　　　　　　　) not.

Patient: What happens if I (**8**　　　　　　　　　) grapefruit juice while taking amlodipine?

Pharmacist: The (**9**　　　　　　) of amlodipine may appear (**10**　　　　　　　) than expected.

Patient: Does it mean my blood pressure (**11**　　　　　　　　　) too (**12**　　　　　　　　　)?

Pharmacist: That's right.

10　Patient: That's scary! I am a scientist and I want to know more about it.

2.ここからは、Alexandraさんからの質問に対して情報提供を行う会話文を作ってみましょう。
情報提供をするために、インターネットや参考文献から情報を検索してまとめましょう。

> Key words: 相互作用　interaction,　～と相互作用する　interact with,
> 　　　　　～と反応する　react with, 柑橘類　citrus fruits, 摂取する　consume

①患者から薬剤師に尋ねること
・アムロジピンとグレープフルーツでどのように相互作用が起きるのかを尋ねる。
・グレープフルーツだけがアムロジピンと相互作用を示すのか、他の柑橘類も摂取できないのか
尋ねる。

②薬剤師が提供する情報
・アムロジピンとグレープフルーツの相互作用のメカニズムを簡単に説明する。
原因となるグレープフルーツの成分　（**13**　　　　　　　　　　　　　　　　　　　　）
原因となるアムロジピンの代謝/動態（**14**　　　　　　　　　　　　　　　　　　　　）
・アムロジピンの服用中に摂取できる、日本にある柑橘類を紹介する。その際、家に持って帰るハンドア
ウトを作り、指し示しながら説明する。
患者に渡すメモ（実際に買い物に行く時に役立つようなものをつくる。）

| Citrus fruits that can be consumed | **15** |
| Citrus fruits to avoid | **16** |

C. A. と **B.** で作成した会話文でロールプレイを行いましょう。その会話から薬歴をSOAP形式
で書いてみましょう。特に、Sでは患者が言ったこと、Aでは薬剤師が患者に言ったことは、
Exercise 2のBのようにキーワードだけではなく、言った通りに英語で書きましょう。

41

Lesson 7

Medication Counseling 2
服薬指導（2）　処方提案・Drug Information（DI）

　　Lesson7では、Lesson6に続いて外国人患者の薬物治療に関しての情報収集と情報提供を行います。外国人患者への服薬指導や受診勧奨、病院のDrug Information（DI）セクションに依頼された医師からの疑問に答えるための情報収集を行います。信頼できる日本語および英語の情報源から情報を収集し、提供してください。英語で書かれた欧州の製品特性概要書（SmPC）は、以下のサイトよりダウンロードできます。

https://www.medicines.org.uk/emc
http://www.mhra.gov.uk/spc-pil/index.htm

Getting to know the genre

Genre: 服薬指導の会話

- **Purpose:**　　　　　　　専門性の高い情報を収集し、患者に必要な情報をわかりやすく提供する
- **Audience***:　　　　　　薬剤師・外国人患者（とその家族）
- **Information:**　　　　　　薬の効果や安全性に関する事象、食物や医薬品との相互作用
- **Language features:**　専門知識を持たない人が理解できる平易な表現、疑問文、接客用語

*ここではParticipants「本書の内容構成と使い方」参照

Checking the terms

(be) admitted	入院する	**expected**	期待される
accumulate	蓄積する	**hip replacement**	人工股関節置換手術
by any chance	もしかして	**insulin injection**	インスリン注射
cholesterol	コレステロール	**perky**	元気な
diabetic	糖尿病の	**plaque formation**	プラーク形成
DVT (deep-vein thrombosis)	深部静脈血栓症	**referral letter**	紹介状
dyslipidaemia[英]	脂質異常症	**run out of**	～が足りなくなる
equivalent to	同等の、同効の	**walk-in clinic**	予約なしで受診できる診療所・医院

42　　*Lesson 7*

Reading the text

あなたは調剤薬局の薬剤師です。あるカナダ人の白人女性がやって来ました。薬のことについて
聞きたいようです。音声を聞いて、自分でも音読しましょう。　　　　　　　（ ◀ｺｺ **Track07-1**）

≪American English≫

Visitor:　　　Excuse me, I wonder if you could help me.

Pharmacist: Certainly. What can I do for you?

Visitor:　　　This is the medicine I take every day for my cholesterol. I was prescribed this medicine
　　　　　　　in Canada. I am about to run out of this medicine and am wondering if I can get this in
5　　　　　　　Japan. By any chance, can I get this medicine over the counter?

Pharmacist: Hmmm. Lovastatin 20 mg.... First of all, all statins are prescription-only in Japan.

Visitor:　　　That is what I expected.

Pharmacist: Secondly, lovastatin is not available in Japan.

Visitor:　　　Oh, no! What should I do? Can I get something similar?

10 Pharmacist: I should think so. Please give me time to make a search.

Visitor:　　　Thank you. I've never visited a physician in Japan. Do I need to make an appointment?

Pharmacist: Not necessarily. Many clinics are walk-in. Would you like me to write a referral letter to a
　　　　　　　physician including the information about the medicine equivalent to lovastatin 20 mg?

Visitor:　　　Oh, that's so kind of you!

15 Pharmacist: In the letter, I'll list some equivalent medicines. You can go to any pharmacy with the
　　　　　　　prescription.

Visitor:　　　I'll come back to this pharmacy with the prescription.

Pharmacist: OK. I'll make sure the letter is ready in about 30 minutes.

➡ Exercise 1

A.

1. この来局者の来局理由は何ですか？

(**1**　　　）

2. この来局者との会話で出てきた2つの問題と、それに対する薬剤師の行動を下の表に日本語で
　 書き入れましょう。

問題点	薬剤師の行動
2	**3**
4	**5**

43

B. 北米ではスタチン系の薬は3段階の強度(intensity)に分類されています。statin intensityを調べて次の表をまとめましょう。そして、医師への紹介状を書くために、lovastatin 20 mgの同効薬で日本にあるもの、この患者に適したものを選んでください。医師と患者に説明できるよう、その薬を選んだ根拠も必要です。lovastatin 20 mgのSmPCが必要な場合は、「lovastatin SmPC」で検索可能です。

Daily dose of statins		
High-intensity (expected LDL reduction 50% or higher)	**Moderate-Intensity** (expected LDL reduction 30 to <50%)	**Low-Intensity** (expected LDL reduction <30%)
1	**2**	**3**

C. 後日、このカナダ人女性が処方箋を持ってあなたの薬局に来ました。あなたが**B.** で選び、紹介状に書いた薬が処方されています。Lesson 6で学んだ初回面談を行ったうえで、今回処方されたlovastatin 20 mgの代替薬について服薬指導を行うシナリオを作ってロールプレイをしましょう。

✏ Exercise 2

あなたは病院薬剤部のDI部門で仕事をしています。糖尿病内科の前田医師から投与量についての問い合わせがありました。患者は、糖尿病で教育入院中のフィリピン人男性Maligayaさんとアフリカ系イギリス人女性のAmershamさんで、脂質異常症の治療が必要と診断されたところです。

A. 前田医師は、ロスバスタチン(rosuvastatin)を処方したいが、人種を考慮して適切な用量を提案して欲しいとのことです。ここでは人種差で投与量に違いのあるロスバスタチンの用量をSmPCをダウンロードして調べてみましょう。

1. 同じ用量のロスバスタチンをMaligayaさん（フィリピン人）とAmershamさん（アフリカ系イギリス人）に投与すると、MaligayaさんのAUC（血中濃度時間曲線下面積）とCmax（最高血中濃度）はAmershamさんと比べてどのような差が出ると予測されますか？
（**1**   ）

2. MaligayaさんとAmershamさんのLDL-C値はそれぞれ250 mg/dLと220 mg/dLです。日本動脈硬化学会による、糖尿病を併発している患者でのLDL-C管理目標値は120 mg/dL未満です。MaligayaさんとAmershamさんのLDL-C目標値を120 mg/dLにして、人種差を考慮してロスバスタチンの適切な投与開始量を決めましょう。

44 *Lesson 7*

	Maligayaさん （フィリピン人）	Amershamさん （アフリカ系イギリス人）
現在のLDL値	250 mg/dL	220 mg/dL
rosuvastatin 適切開始投与量	**2** mg	**3** mg

B. あなたが提供した情報に基づいて、前田医師は２人の患者にロスバスタチンを処方し、２人への服薬指導をあなたに依頼しています。次の３つのポイントは説明しなければならない項目です。まず、英語で書いてみましょう。

①何という名前の、何の治療薬であるか   （**1**   ）
②なぜ治療する必要があるのか   （**2**   ）
③気をつけなければならない副作用   （**3**   ）

薬剤師役と患者役（Maligayaさん及びAmershamさん）に分かれて、それぞれの患者に、服薬指導のロールプレイをやってみましょう。

1. Amershamさんと薬剤師の会話は次のように始めてみましょう。音声も聞きましょう。

（ ◀|| Track07-2）

≪British English≫

Pharmacist: Mrs Amersham, I'm Rei Maruyama, a pharmacist. Dr Maeda asked me to tell you about your new medication. Do you have time now?

Patient: Yes, sure.

Pharmacist: To start with, how are you getting on with the use of the insulin injection?

Patient: I think I'm getting used to it.

Pharmacist: Good. Now, Dr Maeda prescribed a new medicine for dyslipidaemia as your cholesterol level is not good. One of the cholesterols called LDL was much higher than normal.

Patient: Oh, really? What is wrong with high cholesterol?

Pharmacist: Cholesterol that accumulates in your blood vessels causes plaque formation. The plaque narrows your blood vessels, which blocks your blood flow. This is very dangerous as it can cause a heart attack or stroke.

Patient: Oh, no! That's too bad. My father died of a stroke when he was only 58 years old.

ここまでに、すでにポイントの①（適応症）と②（治療の必要性）は言及しています。ロバスタチンが処方されていることと③（副作用）についてはどう説明するか考えてこの会話文を完成させましょう。

2. 次に、Maligayaさんに服薬指導をしましょう。彼は、症状のない脂質異常症に対して病識がなく、新たな薬を飲みたがりません。ポイントの①〜③だけでなく脂質異常症のリスクを丁寧に説明して、納得させる会話文を作りましょう。

45

✏️➡ Exercise 3

Nahla Hamoudaさん は、あなたの薬局によく来局する30代のエジプト人女性です。これまで脂質異常症でシンバスタチン20mgを半年間服用していましたが、3か月くらい前から血圧が高いことを指摘され、1か月前からアムロジピン10mgを服用しています。2週間おきに受診しており、今日もあなたの薬局に次ページの処方箋をもって来局しました。音声を聞きながら、会話の内容を理解しましょう。

(🔊 **Track07-3**)

≪British English≫

Pharmacist: Good afternoon, Nahla. How are you today?

Patient:　　Hmm, not so perky.

Pharmacist: Why is that?

Patient:　　Well, I started to jog and play tennis for my health.

5 Pharmacist: Good for you. So, what's wrong?

Patient:　　My legs, thighs, and arms ache. I'm so tired and don't want to move much.

Pharmacist: That's not good. When did you start jogging and playing tennis?

Patient:　　About one month ago. Since a new medicine for blood pressure was added, I decided to lead a healthy life.

10 Pharmacist: That's a good move. How often do you go jogging and play tennis?

Patient:　　I go jogging with my friend every morning for 1 hour and play tennis with my neighbours three times a week.

Pharmacist: What a big change! However, too much exercise after a long period of no-exercise may be too much for your body.

　Hamoudaさんの筋肉痛の原因で考えられることは何でしょうか？

　単純に、急激な運動による筋肉痛と判断してよいのか、simvastatinのSmPCをダウンロードして調べてみましょう。

1. simvastatin 20mgの副作用で筋肉痛が起きる頻度は何％か？筋肉痛は重要な副作用か？

2. simvastatinとamlodipineの併用によって何が起きる可能性があるか？

3. 副作用なのか、運動による筋肉痛なのか？

　この3つについて検索し、Hamoundaさんにアドバイスをしましょう。

46 *Lesson 7*

右の処方箋の氏名欄には、Hamouda Nahla と記載があります。エジプト人の彼女の正式な名前は、Nahla Mohamed Salah Ibrahim Mousa Hamoudaです。Hamoudaが姓（last name/family name/surname）でNahlaが名（first name/given name）です。これは、名→姓の順に名前が並んでいます。間にある名前はミドルネームと呼ばれるものです。

日本では外国人でも免許証や保険証、その他公式な書類には、日本式に姓→名の順に名前が記載されます。この処方箋ではミドルネームは省略してありますが、公的な文書では、姓→名→ミドルネームの順で記載されます。Nahlaさんのようにミドルネームがいくつもあったり、姓が複数あったり、家族の名前である姓がない国もあります。名前を確認するときは、どれが姓でどれが名なのか、呼びかけるときは、どの名前で呼んで欲しいか尋ねることが大事です。

▶ Applying what you learned

入院に際して、患者は現在服用中の薬を持って入院します。その際、薬剤師はその持参薬をチェックし、服薬状況について聞き取りを行います。

A. Holbornさんはイギリス人男性で股関節置換手術のため入院してきました。次の会話文を音声を聞いて練習し、この後に続く会話文を考えてロールプレイを行ってみましょう。

(🕪 Track 07 -4)

≪British English≫

Pharmacist: Good morning. I'm Kaoru Miyamoto, a pharmacist. You are Mr Holborn and you have just been admitted to this hospital for a hip replacement operation next week. Is this correct?

Patient: Yes, that's right. I'm going to have an operation next week.

5 Pharmacist: I'd like to ask you about your current medications as you may have to stop taking some of them for a while because of the operation.

Patient: Here are the medicines I regularly take. I know which tablet to be taken at what time of the day, but to be honest, I don't know what each tablet is for.

Pharmacist: Do you know why you are taking these medicines?

10 Patient: Yes, I'm diabetic and have hypertension and DVT.* So, I think I'm taking these medicines for them.

Pharmacist: Let me explain which medicine is for what.

47

B. **A.** の会話に出てくるHolbornさんのように自分の飲んでいる薬がよくわかっていない患者さんもいます。巻末Appendix 3Bを参考に以下の薬効別医薬品分類の表を完成させ、説明に利用しましょう。

日本語	英語（専門的）	英語（一般の人が理解できる）
抗不整脈薬	antiarrhythmic	antiarrhythmic, medicine for heart beat
利尿薬	**1**	**2**
降圧薬	**3**	**4**
抗血栓薬、抗血小板薬、抗凝固薬	antithrombotic, **5** , **6**	**7**
血糖降下剤	hypoglycemic agent/drug	**8**
脂質異常症治療薬	antidyslipidaemic[英], antidyslipidemic[米]	cholesterol reducers, cholesterol lowering agent
鎮静薬	**9** tranquiliser[英], tranquilizer[米]	nerve pill, nerve tablet, tranquiliser[英], tranquilizer[米]
抗不安薬	antianxiety agent/drug, anxiolytic	antianxiety
抗うつ薬	antidepressants	antidepressant
睡眠薬	hypnotic	**10**
経口避妊薬	**11**	**12**

48　*Lesson 7*

Lesson 8

Experiment Protocol
実験のプロトコール

　Lesson 8では、科学実験で使用する実験キットのマニュアルを紹介します。実験を簡単に行うために、必要な試薬やカラムなどがあらかじめセットされたキットが多数販売されています。その多くが外国の会社によって開発製造されているため、製品の詳細情報や実験手順（プロトコール）を説明したマニュアルの多くは英語で記載されています。英語で書かれた情報をもとに実験操作が行えるよう必要な情報を取り出す練習をしましょう。

Getting to know the genre

Genre: 実験キットのマニュアル、プロトコール

● Purpose: 　　　　　　実験手順を説明し、指示を与える
● Audience: 　　　　　　このキットを使って実験する研究者・学生
● Information: 　　　　　実験キットの概要と手順
● Language features: 　操作手順を数字で明示、図で視覚化、命令文

Checking the terms

bacterial culture	細菌培養（ここでは大腸菌培養）	**microcentrifuge tube**	マイクロチューブ、微小遠心管
cell lysis buffer	細胞溶解緩衝液	**mix by inverting**	転倒混和
centrifuge	遠心分離する	**neutralize**	中和する
contaminant	汚染物	**opaque**	不透明
debris	デブリ、残骸	**pellet**	小さな塊、ペレット
denatured	変性した	**precipitate**	沈殿物／沈殿する
elution	溶出	**resin**	レジン・樹脂
endotoxin	エンドトキシン*	**robustness**	安定性、耐えうる特性
eukaryotic cell	真核細胞	**supernatant**	上清
flowthrough	フロースルー、通過画分	**yield**	収量

*大腸菌等の細菌の細胞壁構成成分で発熱物質

Reading the text

プラスミドDNAは、大腸菌などの細菌の細胞内で細菌の染色体DNAとは独立して存在し、自律複製する環状の二本鎖DNAです。この性質を利用して、目的とするDNAを組み込んだプラスミド（組み換えプラスミド）を大腸菌内に導入し、適当な培地中で培養・増殖させることによって組み換えプラスミドをもつ大腸菌を大量に調製することができます。プラスミドDNAを大腸菌から抽出する方法の1つがミニプレップ法で、いろいろな手法がありますが、どれも手順が多く時間がかかります。そこで、純度の高いプラスミドDNAを短時間で抽出精製するための商品化されたキットが各社から出されています。ここでは、米国に本社があるPromega社が開発販売している、ミニプレップキットのマニュアルの中から、Description（概要）とProtocol（プロトコール）の部分を読んでみましょう。

PureYield™ Plasmid Miniprep System

Description

The PureYield™ Plasmid Miniprep System isolates high-quality plasmid DNA for use in eukaryotic transfection and in vitro expression experiments. The system provides a rapid method to purify plasmid DNA using a silica-membrane
5　column. Plasmid DNA can be purified in less than 10 minutes, depending on the number of samples processed, greatly reducing the time spent compared to silica resin or other membrane column methods.

The PureYield™Plasmid Miniprep System incorporates a unique Endotoxin Removal Wash to remove protein, RNA and endotoxin contaminants from purified plasmid DNA, improving the robustness of sensitive applications such as eukaryotic transfection, in vitro transcription and coupled in vitro transcription/translation. Purification is achieved
10　without isopropanol precipitation or extensive centrifugation, providing rapid purification of highly concentrated plasmid DNA.

（以下省略）

Protocol

Perform the following procedure at room temperature.

1.　Transfer 600 µl of bacterial culture grown in LB medium to a 1.5 ml microcentrifuge tube.
15　　　**Note**: If you wish to process larger volumes of bacterial culture (up to 3.0 ml), use the protocol provided in section 4.C.
2.　Add 100 µl of Cell Lysis Buffer, and mix by inverting the tube 6 times. The solution should change from opaque to clear blue, indicating complete lysis.
　　　Note: Proceed to Step 3 within 2 minutes. Excessive lysis can result in denatured plasmid DNA. If processing a
20　　　large number of samples, process samples in groups of ten or less. Continue with the next set of ten samples after the first set has been neutralized and mixed thoroughly.
3.　Add 350 µl of cold (4-8° C) Neutralization Solution, and mix thoroughly by inverting the tube.
　　　The sample will turn yellow when neutralization is complete, a yellow precipitate will form. Invert the sample an additional 3 times to ensure complete neutralization.
25　4.　Centrifuge at maximum speed in a centrifuge for 3 minutes.
5.　Transfer the supernatant (~900 µl) to a PureYield™Minicolumn.
　　　Do not disturb the cell debris pellet. For maximum yield, transfer the supernatant with a pipette.
6.　Place the minicolumn into a PureYield™ Collection Tube, and centrifuge at maximum speed in microcentrifuge for 15 seconds.
30　7.　Discard the flowthrough, and place the minicolumn into the same PureYield™ Collection tube.
8.　Add 200 µl of Endotoxin Removal Wash to the minicolumn. Centrifuge at maximum speed in a microcentrifuge for 15 seconds. It is not necessary to empty the PureYield™ Collection Tube.
9.　Add 400 µl of Column Wash Solution to the minicolumn. Centrifuge at maximum speed in a microcentrifuge for 30 seconds.
35　10.　Transfer the minicolumn to a clean 1.5 ml microcentrifuge tube, then add 30 µl of Elution Buffer directly to the minicolumn matrix. Let stand for 1 minute at room temperature.
　　　Notes:
　　　1. Nuclease-free water at neutral pH can also be used to elute DNA.
　　　2. For large plasmids (>10 kb), warm the Elution Buffer to 50° C prior to elution, and increase elution volume to
40　　　　　50 µl. Also incubate the column at room temperature (22-25° C) for 5-10 minutes before proceeding to Step 11.
11.　Centrifuge at maximum speed in a microcentrifuge for 15 seconds to elute the plasmid DNA. Cap the microcentrifuge tube, and store eluted plasmid DNA at -20° C.

50　*Lesson 8*

Exercise 1

本文はDescriptionとProtocolで構成されています。

A. まず、Descriptionの部分を読んで、このキットの概要や利点を理解しましょう。

1. このキットの名称は何ですか？　(**1**　　　　　　　　　　　　　　　　　　　　　　　　)

2. このキットは何をするためのものですか？　It is to～に続く文章で答えましょう。そして、意味を日本語で書きましょう。

　・It is to（**2**　　　　　　　　　　　　　　　　　　　　　　　　　　　　　　　　）

　・（**3**　　　　　　　　　　　　　　　　　　　　　　　　　　　　　）ためのもの

3. 他の方法と比べてこのキットの優れていることは何ですか？　日本語で答えましょう。

　（**4**　　　　　　　　　　　　　　　　　　　　　　　　　　　　　　　　　　　　　）

4. 精製したプラスミドDNAから、タンパク質、RNA、エンドトキシンなどの汚染を除去するために行うステップは何ですか？　本文で該当する部分を抜き出しましょう。

　（**5**　　　　　　　　　　　　　　　　　　　　　　　　　　　　　　　　　　　　　）

5. 3.で答えたステップの利点（**4**）を、This step improves～に続く文章で答えましょう。

　This step improves（**6**　　　　　　　　　　　　　　　　　　　　　　　　　　　　　）

B. Protocol (Step 1～11) を読んで実験手順を確認しましょう。

　Step 1, 2を読んで答えましょう。

1. （**7**　　　　）µlの菌培養液に（**8**　　　　　　）µlのCell Lysis Bufferを加えて溶解する。

2. 菌の溶解が完了すると、溶液の状態はどのように変化するはずですか？　該当部分を英語で書き抜きましょう。次に日本語で説明しましょう。

　・（**9**　　　　　　　　　　　　　　　　　　　　　　　　　　　　　　　　　　　　）

　・溶液が、（**10**　　　　　　　　　　）から（**11**　　　　　　　　　　）に変化するはずである。

3. サンプル数が多い場合は、1グループ（**12**　　　　　　　　）サンプル以下に分けて、最初のグループの（**13**　　　　　　　　　）と（**14**　　　　　　　　　　）を行ってから、次のサンプルグループの処理を行う。

　Step 3, 4を読んで答えましょう。

4. 中和が完了すると、サンプルの状態はどのように変化するはずですか？　英語で書き抜きましょう。次に日本語で説明しましょう。

　・（**15**　　　　　　　　　　　　　　　　　　　　　　　　　　　　　　　　　　　）

　・中和が完了すると、サンプルは（**16**　　　　　　）になり、（**17**　　　　　　　）ができる。

　Step 5～11を読んで、本文から該当する部分を書き抜きましょう。

5. PureYield™ Minicolumnには何µlまでの上清を移すことができますか？　（**18**　　　　　）

6. 溶出に使うElution Bufferの代わりに何を使うことができますか？　（**19**　　　　　）

7. 室温とは何℃のことですか？　（**20**　　　　　　　　　　　　　　　　　　　）

51

Exercise 2

次の文章は、Reading the textで読んだ詳細なProtocol（Complete Protocol）の要点を実際に実験をする時に参照できるように、イラスト入りでまとめたQuick Protocolです。Quick Protocolの"DNA Purification by Centrifugation"のStep 1 ～ Step 11は、Complete ProtocolのStep 1 ～ Step 11に対応していますので見比べてみましょう。

PureYield™ Plasmid Miniprep System

INSTRUCTIONS FOR USE OF PRODUCTS A1220, A1221, A1222 AND A1223

Quick PROTOCOL

Solution Preparation

Before lysing cells and purifying DNA, prepare the Column Wash Solution by adding ethanol. Cap tightly after addition. See Technical Bulletin #TB374 for detailed instructions.

DNA Purification by Centrifugation

Prepare Lysate

1. Add 600µl of bacterial culture to a 1.5ml microcentrifuge tube.
   Note: For higher yields and purity use the alternative protocol below to harvest and process up to 3ml of bacterial culture.

2. Add 100µl of Cell Lysis Buffer (Blue), and mix by inverting the tube 6 times.

3. Add 350µl of cold (4–8°C) Neutralization Solution, and mix thoroughly by inverting.

4. Centrifuge at maximum speed in a microcentrifuge for 3 minutes.

5. Transfer the supernatant (~900µl) to a PureYield™ Minicolumn without disturbing the cell debris pellet.

6. Place the minicolumn into a Collection Tube, and centrifuge at maximum speed in a microcentrifuge for 15 seconds.

7. Discard the flowthrough, and place the minicolumn into the same Collection Tube.

Wash

8. Add 200µl of Endotoxin Removal Wash (ERB) to the minicolumn. Centrifuge at maximum speed in a microcentrifuge for 15 seconds.

9. Add 400µl of Column Wash Solution (CWC) to the minicolumn. Centrifuge at maximum speed in a microcentrifuge for 30 seconds.

Elute

10. Transfer the minicolumn to a clean 1.5ml microcentrifuge tube, then add 30µl of Elution Buffer or nuclease-free water directly to the minicolumn matrix. Let stand for 1 minute at room temperature.

11. Centrifuge for 15 seconds to elute the plasmid DNA. Cap the microcentrifuge tube, and store eluted plasmid DNA at –20°C.

Alternative Protocol for Larger Culture Volumes

1. Centrifuge 1.5ml of bacterial culture for 30 seconds at maximum speed in a microcentrifuge. Discard the supernatant.

2. Add an additional 1.5ml of bacterial culture to the same tube and repeat Step 1.

3. Add 600µl of TE buffer or water to the cell pellet, and resuspend completely.

4. Proceed to Step 2 of the standard protocol above.

For complete protocol information see Technical Bulletin #TB374, available at: www.promega.com/tbs

ORDERING / TECHNICAL INFORMATION:
www.promega.com • Phone 608-274-4330 or 800-356-9526 • Fax 608-277-2601

© 2008, 2009 Promega Corporation. All Rights Reserved.

Printed in USA. Revised 8/09
Part #9FB093

Promega

Illustration labels (a–k):

- **a**
- **b** Lyse cells. Neutralize.
- **c** Centrifuge.
- **d** Transfer supernatant to PureYield™ Minicolumn.
- **e** Place PureYield™ Minicolumn in a Collection Tube. Centrifuge.
- **f** Add Endotoxin Removal Wash.
- **g** Centrifuge.
- **h** Add Column Wash Solution.
- **i** Centrifuge.
- **j** Transfer PureYield™ Minicolumn to a clean 1.5ml microcentrifuge tube. Add Elution Buffer or water.
- **k** Centrifuge to elute DNA.

※ 実験手順を撮影した動画を視聴、ダウンロードできます。
https://www.promega.jp/resources/protocols/technical-bulletins/101/pureyield-plasmid-miniprep-system-protocol/

52 *Lesson 8*

A. Quick Protocolのイラスト**a〜k**は、それぞれstep 1〜step 11のどれに対応していますか？　下の表を埋めましょう。

イラスト	step
a	1
b	**1**
c	**2**
d	**3**
e	**4**
f	8
g	**5**
h	**6**
i	**7**
j	**8**
k	11

B. このキットを使って自分が実験することを想定して、Quick Protocolを元に日本語のプロトコールをフローチャートで書いてみましょう。

培養した大腸菌600 μl
↓
1 _____
↓
2 _____
↓
3 _____
↓
4 _____
↓
5 _____
↓
6 _____
↓
7 _____
↓
15秒遠心分離機にかけプラスミドDNAを溶出

C. Complete Protocolにのみ書かれていて、Quick Protocolに書かれていないのはどのような情報ですか？　Complete ProtocolとQuick ProtocolのStep 1〜Step 11のうち、次の3つのStepでプロトコールを見比べて日本語で書きましょう。

Step 2:　(**1** 　　　　　　　　　　　　　　　　　　　　　　　　　　　　　)
　　　　　(**2** 　　　　　　　　　　　　　　　　　　　　　　　　　　　　　)
Step 3:　(**3** 　　　　　　　　　　　　　　　　　　　　　　　　　　　　　)
　　　　　(**4** 　　　　　　　　　　　　　　　　　　　　　　　　　　　　　)
Step 5:　(**5** 　　　　　　　　　　　　　　　　　　　　　　　　　　　　　)

　このように、Complete Protocolには、Quick Protocolにない詳しい実験の条件などが示されています。そのような文章は、指示文で使われる命令形だけではなく、状態を説明する現在形や、状態の変化を説明する未来形が使われます。また、"Note"という表示をつけることで注意を惹きつけるなど、書き方に工夫がなされています。このような違いを、Complete ProtocolのStep 2やStep 3を見て確認しましょう。

Exercise 3

A. 実験の操作を表現する代表的な動詞が以下の選択肢に含まれています。空欄に入る単語を選び、適切な形に変えて書き入れましょう。音声を聞いて確認しましょう。（ ⁻⁝⁾⁾ **Track08-1**）

centrifuge	dilute	discard	incubate	invert	place	replace

1. チューブを傾けて溶液を転倒混和する。

   Mix the solution by（ **1**　　　　）the tube.

2. ペレットを作るためにマイクロチューブを遠心分離機にかける。

   （ **2**　　　　）the microcentrifuge tube to make a pellet.

3. 上清は捨てて、ペレットは取っておく。

   （ **3**　　　　）the supernatant and keep the pellet.

4. 10x buffer 1容量を9容量の水で薄めて溶液を調整する。

   Prepare the solution by（ **4**　　　）1 volume of 10x buffer with 9 volumes of water.

5. 細胞培養培地を新しい培地と交換する。

   （ **5**　　　　）the cell culture medium with a new medium.

6. マイクロチューブをチューブ立てに静置する。

   （ **6**　　　　）the microcentrifuge tubes in the tube stand.

7. 細菌をLBプレート上で、37°Cで一晩培養する。

   Bacteria are grown on an LB plate by（ **7**　　　　）at 37°C overnight.

B. プロトコールによく出てくる表現です。空欄に入る適切な語を選択肢の中から選んで、文章を完成させましょう。同じ語を複数回使えます。音声を聞いて確認しましょう。

（ ⁻⁝⁾⁾ **Track08-2**）

at	for	in	on	to	until	up	with

1. To lyse the cells, suspend the cell pellet（ **1**　）lysis buffer A（ **2**　）a pipette.

2. Centrifuge the microcentrifuge tube（ **3**　）4°C（ **4**　）3 minutes.

3. Place the sample（ **5**　）ice.

4. Rinse the beaker（ **6**　）deionized water*.　*脱イオン水

5. Make 100 µl aliquots** of new reagent B and store（ **7**　）the -80°C freezer（ **8**　）use.

   **分注

6. This machine heats（ **9**　　）（ **10**　　）100°C.

7. The sample is stable（ **11**　）solution C（ **12**　）4 weeks.

54 *Lesson 8*

C. プロトコールに従って実験を行なった後、その方法や手順を論文に書く際には、無生物主語を使い、過去形の受動態で書きます。次の命令形の文章を、下の例にならって書き換えましょう。

例：Pour 10-50 mL of overnight culture into a conical tube.

→ Ten to fifty milliliters of overnight culture was poured into a conical tube.

1 Transfer 600 µL of bacterial culture grown in LB medium to a 1.5 mL microcentrifuge tube.

2 Add 100 µL of Cell Lysis Buffer, and mix by inverting the tube 6 times.

3 Mix thoroughly by inverting the tube.

4 Centrifuge at maximum speed in a microcentrifuge for 3 minutes.

5 Cap the microcentrifuge tube, and store the eluted plasmid DNA at –20℃.

✏ Applying what you learned

自分の研究に有用なキットのマニュアルやプロトコールをインターネットで検索してダウンロードし、complete protocolまたはquick protocolから日本語のquick protocolをつくってみましょう。適宜、イラストを入れるとわかりやすくなるでしょう。

参考（キットの例）:

QIAquick PCR purification Kit (QIAGEN)

Direct-zol RNA Miniprep Kit (ZYMO Research)

BigDye® X Terminator® Purification Kit (ThermoFisher Scientific)

Apo-Direct Apoptosis Detection Kit (ThermoFisher Scientific)

※マニュアルには、Complete Protocolだけではなく、実験法の原理、使用上の注意、キットに入っているもののリスト、実験前に用意するもの、トラブルシューティング（思うような結果が得られなかった時の解決策）など、必要に応じて読むべき情報が記載されています。マニュアル（Manual）は、キットを製造販売している会社によってHandbookやUser Guideなどとよばれています。Complete ProtocolをFull Protocol と呼ぶこともありますし、Quick Protocolも、Quick Reference, Protocol-at-a-glance, Protocol Overview, Experimental Overviewなど、会社によっていろいろな呼び方があります。

Lesson 9

Research Article 1: Title, Abstract
臨床試験の原著論文を読む(1)　表題と要旨

　Lesson 9〜13では論文の読み方を学習します。研究で得られた最新の知見は、学術論文としてNatureやScienceなどの商業誌や学会が発行する学会誌に掲載されることで世界に発表されます。ここで扱う論文は、米国医師会が発行するJAMA（The Journal of American Medical Association）という総合医学雑誌に掲載された原著論文（original contribution）で、ALLHATと名付けられた大規模臨床試験の主な結果を報告しています。Lesson 9ではまず、Title（表題）とAbstract（要旨）について学びましょう。

Getting to know the genre

Genre: 原著論文の「表題」・「要旨」

- **Purpose:**　　　　　論文本文の概要を提供する
- **Audience:**　　　　　医療専門家、研究者
- **Information:**　　　　研究の背景、目的、デザイン、結果、結論の簡潔な記述
- **Language features:**　IMRAD*による構成、専門用語、図表や引用は含まない

*IMRAD: Introduction, Methods, Results, and Discussion

Checking the terms

all-cause mortality	全死因死亡	intervention	介入
combined	複合した	mean	平均
confidence interval (CI)	信頼区間	morbidity	罹患率
context	背景	mortality	死亡率
establish	確立する	objective	目的
event	イベント、事象	optimal	最適な
fatal	致死的な	outcome	転帰、結果
first-step therapy	一次治療	participant	参加者、被験者
follow-up	追跡期間	primary	主要な
hospitalization[※]	入院	relative risk (RR)	相対危険度
incidence	発生率	secondary	副次的な
intent-to-treat	ITT（解析方法の1つ）	(clinical) trial	臨床試験

56　*Lesson 9*

Reading the text

Major Outcomes in High-Risk Hypertensive Patients Randomized to Angiotensin-Converting Enzyme Inhibitor or Calcium Channel Blocker vs Diuretic （ •))| Track09-1）
The Antihypertensive and Lipid-Lowering Treatment to Prevent Heart Attack Trial (ALLHAT)

5 **Abstract**

Context Antihypertensive therapy is well established to reduce hypertension-related morbidity and mortality, but the optimal first-step therapy is unknown.

Objective To determine whether treatment with a calcium channel blocker
10 or an angiotensin-converting enzyme inhibitor lowers the incidence of coronary heart disease (CHD) or other cardiovascular disease (CVD) events vs treatment with a diuretic.

Design The Antihypertensive and Lipid-Lowering Treatment to Prevent Heart Attack Trial (ALLHAT), a randomized, double-blind, active-controlled
15 clinical trial conducted from February 1994 through March 2002.

Setting and Participants A total of 33 357 participants aged 55 years or older with hypertension and at least 1 other CHD risk factor from 623 North American centers.

Interventions Participants were randomly assigned to receive chlorthalidone,
20 12.5 to 25 mg/d (n = 15 255); amlodipine, 2.5 to 10 mg/d (n = 9048); or lisinopril, 10 to 40 mg/d (n = 9054) for planned follow-up of approximately 4 to 8 years.

Main Outcome Measures The primary outcome was combined fatal CHD or nonfatal myocardial infarction, analyzed by intent-to-treat. Secondary
25 outcomes were all-cause mortality, stroke, combined CHD (primary outcome, coronary revascularization, or angina with hospitalization), and combined CVD (combined CHD, stroke, treated angina without hospitalization, heart failure [HF], and peripheral arterial disease).

Results Mean follow-up was 4.9 years. The primary outcome occurred in
30 2956 participants, with no difference between treatments. Compared with chlorthalidone (6-year rate, 11.5%), the relative risks (RRs) were 0.98 (95% CI, 0.90-1.07) for amlodipine (6-year rate, 11.3%) and 0.99 (95% CI, 0.91-1.08) for lisinopril (6-year rate, 11.4%). Likewise, all-cause mortality did not differ between groups. Five-year systolic blood pressures were significantly
35 higher in the amlodipine (0.8 mm Hg, P = .03) and lisinopril (2 mm Hg, P<.001) groups compared with chlorthalidone, and 5-year diastolic blood pressure was significantly lower with amlodipine (0.8 mm Hg, P<.001). For amlodipine vs chlorthalidone, secondary outcomes were similar except for a higher 6-year rate of HF with amlodipine (10.2% vs 7.7%; RR, 1.38; 95%
40 CI, 1.25-1.52). For lisinopril vs chlorthalidone, lisinopril had higher 6-year rates of combined CVD (33.3% vs 30.9%; RR, 1.10; 95% CI, 1.05-1.16); stroke (6.3% vs 5.6%; RR, 1.15; 95% CI, 1.02-1.30); and HF (8.7% vs 7.7%; RR, 1.19; 95% CI, 1.07-1.31).

Conclusion Thiazide-type diuretics are superior in preventing 1 or more
45 major forms of CVD and are less expensive. They should be preferred for first-step antihypertensive therapy.

Angiotensin-Converting Enzyme Inhibitor
アンジオテンシン変換酵素阻害薬

Calcium Channel Blocker
カルシウムチャネル遮断薬

Diuretic　利尿薬

Lipid-Lowering
脂質を低下させる

Heart Attack　心臓発作

coronary heart disease (CHD)
冠動脈心疾患

cardiovascular disease (CVD)
心血管疾患

myocardial infarction
心筋梗塞

stroke　脳卒中

coronary revascularization
冠動脈再灌流

angina　狭心症

heart failure [HF]　心不全

peripheral arterial disease
末梢動脈疾患

systolic blood pressure
収縮期血圧

diastolic blood pressure
拡張期血圧

thiazide-type diuretic
サイアザイド系利尿薬

Exercise 1

学術論文の表題にはその論文のキーワードが含まれているので、表題を見ただけで論文本文の骨子が理解できます。この論文のキーワードを表題に含まれる語から見つけ出し、英語のまま下の表の空欄に当てはめて整理しましょう。

Major Outcomes in High-Risk Hypertensive Patients Randomized to Angiotensin-Converting Enzyme Inhibitor or Calcium Channel Blocker vs Diuretic

対象患者は?	1	
使われた薬は?	作用機序による分類名	薬剤名
	2	lisinopril
	3	amlodipine
	4 （比較対照薬*）	chlorthalidone
臨床試験のデザインを表すキーワード**	5	

*比較対照薬は vs（versus：対）の後に記されています。
**臨床試験のデザインを表すキーワードは p.61 の表を参照してください。

Exercise 2

Abstract（要旨）は Summary と呼ばれることもあり、論文本文の概要を示します。この論文の本文は、Introduction*（序論）、Methods**（研究方法）、Results（結果）、Comment***（考察）と呼ばれる4つのセクションから成り、それぞれ下記の役割を持っています。

論文の4セクションの役割

Introduction　研究の背景、範囲、目的を提示する
Methods　　　目的を達成するために何をしたか、研究方法を明記する
Results　　　　研究結果をデータと共に提示する
Discussion***　結果を解釈し、論点に対する解答を与えて結論を示す

*この論文では序論の冒頭に Introduction という見出しは印字されていません。
**Methods（方法）は Materials and Methods, Procedures などの呼び名が使われることもあります。
***この論文では Comment（考察）という呼び名が使われています。

　この論文の Abstract には上記の4セクションに対応する見出しが付けられ、内容がわかりやすく整理されています。このようにセクション分けされた Abstract を Structured Abstract（構造化要旨）といいます。

58　*Lesson 9*

A. 下表はAbstractの見出しが論文の4セクションとどう対応しているかを示しています。対応関係を確認しながらAbstractの見出しの英語表記を記入しましょう。

論文の4セクション	対応するAbstractのセクション	
Introduction	**1**	（背景）
	2	（目的）
Methods	**3**	（試験デザイン）
	4	（設定と参加者）
	5	（介入）
	6	（主要評価項目）
Results	**7**	（結果）
Comment	**8**	（結論）

B. 論文本文を読む前にAbstractのContext（背景）、Objective（目的）、Conclusion（結論）を読むと、研究の目的と結論を先取りすることができます。以下にAbstractの各セクションの文をスラッシュ（斜線）で区切って示していますので、区切られた各部分が文法的に何を示しているか文の構造を確認しながら、英語のまま解答欄に記入しましょう。

次に、対応する日本語訳の空欄に適切な言葉を埋めて内容を理解しましょう。

Context Antihypertensive therapy/ is well established/ to reduce hypertension-related morbidity and mortality,// but/ the optimal first-step therapy/ is unknown.

主語1：**1**	動詞部1：**2**	
どのような点で：**3**		but
主語2：**4**	動詞部2：**5**	

（**6**　　　　　　　　　　　）は、（**7**　　　　　　　　　　　　　　　　　　　　）
させる事が実証されているが（**8**　　　　　　　　　　　　　　　　）は不明である。

59

Objective To determine whether /treatment with a calcium channel blocker or an angiotensin-converting enzyme inhibitor/ lowers/ the incidence of coronary heart disease (CHD)/ or other cardiovascular disease (CVD) events/ vs treatment with a diuretic.

```
To determine whether … ：～かどうかを確かめる/検証すること*
主語：9
動詞：10
目的語 1：11                                              or
目的語 2：12
何と比較して：13
```

*Objectiveの文は「… すること」という長い名詞句になっており、whether 以下がdetermineの意味上の目的語になっています。

（14   ）による治療が、

（15   ）による治療と比較して、

（16   ）を低減するかどうかを検証すること。

Conclusion Thiazide-type diuretics/ are/ superior/ in preventing 1 or more major forms of CVD //and are /less expensive/.

```
主語： 17
動詞 1：18
補語 1：19
どういう点で：20                                          and
動詞 2：21
補語 2：22
```

（23   ）は、（24   ）
という点で優れており、また（25   ）

They/ should be preferred/ for first-step antihypertensive therapy/.

```
主語：They
動詞：26
どのような使い方で：27
```

それらは、（28   ）されるべきである。
主語のtheyは何を指す？（29   ）

60 *Lesson 9*

C. Designには、この試験の名称であるALLHATに続いて試験デザインを表す表現が示されています。試験デザインを表す用語は臨床試験の論文を読む際に押さえておくべきキーワードのひとつです。下の表を参照しながらALLHATの試験デザインを確認しましょう。

Randomized,　double-blind,　active-controlled clinical trial
（ **1**　　　　）（ **2**　　　　）（ **3**　　　　）　臨床試験

臨床試験のデザインを表すキーワード

無作為化の有無	randomized　無作為化		non-randomized　非無作為化	
盲検化	double-blind/masked	二重盲検(研究者も参加者も治療内容を知らない)		
	single-blind	単盲検(参加者は治療内容を知らない)		
	unblinded, open-label	非盲検(治療内容がマスクされていない)		
比較対照群	controlled, comparative	比較対照群をおいた		
	active/positive-controlled	実薬対照		
	placebo-controlled	プラセボ(偽薬)対照		
	uncontrolled	無対照		
参加施設数	multicenter (multicentre)　多施設共同		single-center　単一施設	

　この論文のタイトルにはrandomizedというキーワードのみ記されています。臨床試験のうちRandomized Controlled Trial（無作為化比較対照試験：RCT）はEvidence-Based Medicine（EBM）の根拠となり、治療ガイドラインなどにその結果が反映されます。

D. Intervention（介入）では、この臨床試験で比較される治療群（treatment arm/group）が記載されています。各治療群の薬剤名、投与量、人数を下の図にまとめましょう。

治療群（薬剤名）	投与量	人数*
chlorthalidone	**1**	**2**
3	2.5-10 mg/day	**4**
5	**6**	9,054

randomization 無作為化

*各治療群の人数を足すとSetting and Participantsに記載されている参加者数合計(33,357人)と一致することがわかります。

E. Main Outcome Measures（主要評価項目）は、primary outcome（主要転帰）と secondary outcomes（副次的転帰）にわけて記述されています。

1. 主要転帰（primary outcome）を説明する文を英語のまま書き出しましょう。

```
┌──────────────────────────────────────────────┐
│                                              │
│                                              │
│                                              │
│                                              │
└──────────────────────────────────────────────┘
```

2. 副次的転帰（secondary outcomes）を示す文を英語のまま書き出しましょう。

```
┌──────────────────────────────────────────────┐
│                                              │
│                                              │
│                                              │
│                                              │
└──────────────────────────────────────────────┘
```

※評価項目の詳細はLesson 11のp.77（Outcomes）に示されていますので確認しましょう。

F. Results（結果）では、主要転帰や副次的転帰について治療群間に差が認められたかどうかを示す比較表現が多用されます。特に、その差が統計学的に有意であったときにはsignificant（形容詞）やsignificantly（副詞）という語が用いられます。

Resultsに関する以下の文を日本語に訳して内容を理解しましょう。

1. Mean follow-up was 4.9 years.（**1**   ）

2. The primary outcome occurred in 2956 participants, with no difference between treatments.
   （**2**   ）

3. Likewise, all-cause mortality did not differ between groups.
   （**3**   ）

4. Five-year systolic blood pressures were significantly higher in the amlodipine and lisinopril groups compared with chlorthalidone, and 5-year diastolic blood pressure was significantly lower with amlodipine.
   5年後の（**4**   ）血圧は（**5**   ）、
   5年後の（**6**   ）血圧は（**7**   ）

5. For amlodipine vs chlorthalidone, secondary outcomes were similar except for a higher 6-year rate of HF with amlodipine.
   アムロジピンとクロルサリドンの比較では、（**8**   ）
   ことを除き、副次的転帰は（**9**   ）

62   *Lesson 9*

6. For lisinopril vs chlorthalidone, lisinopril had higher 6-year rates of combined CVD, stroke, and HF.

リシノプリルとクロルサリドンの比較では、(🔟

）

✏️ Applying what you learned

以下の論文タイトルについて、**1** 検討した治療法（とその比較対照）、**2** 対象疾患 / 参加者集団、**3** 評価項目、**4** 試験デザインを表すキーワードを抜き出しましょう。

A. The Journal of American Medical Association (JAMA)

Effect of Antihypertensive Agents on Cardiovascular Events in Patients with Coronary Disease and Normal Blood Pressure The CAMELOT Study: A Randomized Controlled Trial

1 検討した治療法等

2 対象疾患 / 参加者集団

3 評価項目

4 試験デザイン

B. The British Medical Journal (BMJ)

Impact of inhalational versus intravenous anaesthesia on early delirium and long-term survival in elderly patients after cancer surgery: study protocol of a multicentre, open-label, and randomised controlled trial

1 検討した治療法等

2 対象疾患 / 参加者集団

3 評価項目

4 試験デザイン

C. The Lancet

Safety, tolerability, and immunogenicity of two Zika virus DNA vaccine candidates in healthy adults: randomised, open-label, phase 1 clinical trials

1 検討した治療法等

2 対象疾患 / 参加者集団

3 評価項目

4 試験デザイン

D. Cardiovascular Diabetology

Efficacy and safety of monotherapy with the novel sodium/glucose cotransporter-2 inhibitor tofogliflozin in Japanese patients with type 2 diabetes mellitus: a combined Phase 2 and 3 randomized, placebo-controlled, double-blind, parallel-group comparative study

1 検討した治療法等

2 対象疾患 / 参加者集団

3 評価項目

4 試験デザイン

E. Clinical Opthalmology

A study protocol for evaluating the efficacy and safety of skin electrical stimulation for Leber hereditary optic neuropathy: a single-arm, open-label, non-randomized prospective exploratory study

1 検討した治療法等

2 対象疾患 / 参加者集団

3 評価項目

4 試験デザイン

64 *Lesson 9*

Lesson *10*

Research Article 2: Introduction
臨床試験の原著論文を読む（2）　序論

　Introduction（序論）は、論文本体の最初のセクションで、その研究がいかに重要で必要なのかを説明する役割があります。まず、その研究領域の社会での位置づけや重要性を示し、その領域で今までに行われた研究（先行研究）を紹介し、未解決のニーズや問題を提起し、それを解決するために今回どのような研究をしたかを述べるという流れで話が絞り込まれます。この流れを意識して、特徴的な表現や時制に気を付けながら読み進めましょう。

Getting to know the genre

Genre: 原著論文の「序論」
- **Purpose:** 　　　　　　　研究の重要性と研究目的を伝える
- **Audience:** 　　　　　　 医療専門家、研究者
- **Information:** 　　　　　研究の重要性、先行研究、未解決の事柄、研究目的
- **Language features:** 広い領域から論点の事柄に情報を絞り込む流れ、時制の使い分け

Checking the terms

agent	薬剤	regarding	〜について
annually	1年間に	relative	相対的な
complication	合併症	represent	代表する
considerable	相当の	sample size	サンプルサイズ（被験者数）
decade	10年	sponsor	資金提供する
document	立証する	study	試験 ※trialと同義
early termination	早期中止		
pharmacotherapy	薬物療法	substantially	大幅に
present	示す	uncertain	不確かな
previously	以前に	usual care	通常治療
primarily	主に		

65

Reading the text

Treatment and complications among the 50 to 60 million people in the United States with hypertension are estimated to cost $37 billion annually, with antihypertensive drug costs alone accounting for an estimated $15.5 billion per year. Antihypertensive drug therapy substantially reduces the risk
5 of hypertension-related morbidity and mortality. However, the optimal choice for initial pharmacotherapy of hypertension is uncertain.

Earlier clinical trials documented the benefit of lowering blood pressure (BP) using primarily thiazide diuretics or β-blockers. After these studies, several newer classes of antihypertensive agents (ie, angiotensin-converting
10 enzyme [ACE] inhibitors, calcium channel blockers [CCBs], α-adrenergic blockers, and more recently angiotensin-receptor blockers) became available. Over the past decade, major placebo-controlled trials have documented that ACE inhibitors and CCBs reduce cardiovascular events in individuals with hypertension. However, their relative value compared with
15 older, less expensive agents remains unclear. There has been considerable uncertainty regarding effects of some classes of antihypertensive drugs on risk of coronary heart disease (CHD). The relative benefit of various agents in high-risk hypertensive subgroups such as older patients, black patients, and patients with diabetes also needed to be established.
20 The Antihypertensive and Lipid-Lowering Treatment to Prevent Heart Attack Trial (ALLHAT), a randomized, double-blind, multicenter clinical trial sponsored by the National Heart, Lung, and Blood Institute, was designed to determine whether the occurrence of fatal CHD or nonfatal myocardial infarction is lower for high-risk patients with hypertension
25 treated with a CCB (represented by amlodipine), an ACE inhibitor (represented by lisinopril), or an α-blocker (represented by doxazosin), each compared with diuretic treatment (represented by chlorthalidone). Chlorthalidone was found to be superior to doxazosin and was previously reported after early termination of the doxazosin arm of the trial. Secondary
30 outcomes included all-cause mortality, stroke, and other cardiovascular disease (CVD) events. A lipid-lowering subtrial was designed to determine whether lowering cholesterol with 3-hydroxy-3-methylglutaryl coenzyme A reductase inhibitor (pravastatin) compared with usual care reduced all-cause mortality in a moderately hypercholesterolemic subset of ALLHAT
35 participants. To evaluate differences in CVD effects of the various first-step drugs, ALLHAT was designed with a large sample size (9000-15000 participants/intervention arm) and long follow-up (4-8 years). This study presents results of the amlodipine and lisinopril vs chlorthalidone comparisons on major CVD outcomes.

β-blockers　β遮断薬

α-adrenergic blockers
　αアドレナリン遮断薬

angiotensin-receptor blockers
　アンジオテンシン受容体遮断薬

National Heart, Lung, and Blood Institute
　国立心肺血液研究所(米国)

lipid-lowering subtrial
　脂質低下薬の効果を検討したALLHAT試験のサブ試験

3-hydroxy-3-methylglutaryl coenzyme A reductase inhibitor
　3-ヒドロキシ-3-メチルグルタリル補酵素A還元酵素阻害薬(HMG-CoA還元酵素阻害薬)

66 *Lesson 10*

Exercise 1

冒頭に示したように、Introductionには流れがあり、これは科学的実証研究の論文では学問分野を問わず共通のものです。このように、特定のジャンルに含まれる情報の流れを「ムーブ」と呼びます。Introductionのムーブは次の4つです。

背景ムーブ	その論文が扱う研究領域の社会における位置づけと重要性、研究分野の歴史的背景、現状を示す。重要な事柄や概念の定義、説明などが含まれる。
先行研究ムーブ	その研究領域で過去に行われた研究（先行研究）により既に解明されている事柄や知見を紹介する。
ギャップムーブ	先行研究で解明された事柄を受けて、「しかしながら…はまだ不明である、未解決である」と問題点を指摘し、医療上のニーズとの間にギャップが存在することを指摘する。「だから私達はそのギャップを埋めるために今回このような研究を行った」と、本研究ムーブに橋渡しをする。
本研究ムーブ	ギャップムーブで指摘された研究動機を踏まえてどのような研究を行ったのか、その研究目的と範囲を示す。

ムーブを特定することができればIntroductionはとても読みやすくなります。各ムーブには汎用される定型的な表現があり、ムーブを特定するヒントとなることから、本書ではそれをHint Expressions (HE)と呼ぶことにします。以下に各ムーブに含まれるHEの特徴と動詞の時制がまとめられています。また、論文本文から抜き出したHE（下線部）を含む文を示していますので、意味を確認しながら空欄を埋めましょう。次に、前ページに示されているIntroduction全体を読んで、どこからどこまでが各ムーブに該当するか考えて、文を区切りましょう。

A. 背景ムーブのHint Expressions

特徴	動詞の時制
研究分野の特定とその重要性や現状を強調する表現、大きい数字など	現在形または現在完了形

1. Treatment and complications among the <u>50 to 60 million people</u> in the United States with hypertension <u>are estimated to cost $37 billion annually</u>, with antihypertensive drug costs alone accounting for an estimated <u>$15.5 billion per year</u>.

　米国における高血圧患者（**1**　　　　　）人の治療や合併症には、年間（**2**　　　　　）ドルの費用がかかると見積もられており、高血圧治療薬だけで年間（**3**　　　　　）ドルを占めると概算されている。

2. Antihypertensive drug therapy <u>substantially reduces</u> the risk of hypertension-related morbidity and mortality.

　高血圧の薬物療法は、高血圧関連の（**4**　　　　　）や（**5**　　　　　）を大幅に低減する。

67

B. 先行研究ムーブのHint Expressions

特徴	動詞の時制
先行研究を指す語や文献番号の記載、既に立証されていることを示すdocumentedなどの表現	現在完了形または過去形

1. Earlier clinical trials documented the benefit of lowering blood pressure (BP) using primarily thiazide diuretics or β-blockers.

（**1**⃣　　　　　　　　　　　　　　　　　　　　）は、主にサイアザイド系利尿薬またはβ-遮断薬を使用して血圧（BP）を下げることの（**2**⃣　　　　　　　　　　　　　　　　）

2. Over the past decade, major placebo-controlled trials have documented that ACE-inhibitors and CCBs reduce cardiovascular events in individuals with hypertension.

過去10年間にわたり、（**3**⃣　　　　　　　　　　　　　　　　）は、ACE阻害薬とCCBが高血圧を持つ人々における心血管系イベントを低減することを（**4**⃣　　　　　　　　　　　）

C. ギャップムーブのHint Expressions

特徴	動詞の時制
However（しかしながら）、不確かな事柄の存在を示すunknownやuncertain、さらなる研究の必要性を示唆するnecessaryやneedなどの表現	現在形または現在完了形

1. However, their relative value compared with older, less expensive agents remains unclear.

しかしながら、（**1**⃣　　　　　　　　　　　　　　　　　　　）は未だ不明である。

2. There has been considerable uncertainty regarding effects of some classes of antihypertensive drugs on risk of coronary heart disease (CHD).

（**2**⃣　　　　　　　　　　　　　　　　　　　　　　　　　　　　　）についてはかなり不確実である。

3. The relative benefit of various agents in high-risk hypertensive subgroups such as older patients, black patients, and patients with diabetes also needed to be established.

（**3**⃣　　　　　　　　　　　　　　　　　　）など、高リスクの高血圧患者サブグループにおける（**4**⃣　　　　　　　　　　　）についても確立される必要がある。

68　*Lesson 10*

D. 本研究ムーブの Hint Expressions

特徴	動詞の時制
「この研究」(this study, present researchなど)、「この論文」(this article, paperなど)、「我々は」(we)などの表現、研究目的を示す副詞句(to/in order to …)、研究内容(治療群、評価項目など)を示す表現	現在形または過去形

1. <u>To evaluate</u> differences in CVD effects of the various first-step drugs, ALLHAT <u>was designed with</u> a large sample size (9,000-15,000 participants/intervention arm) and long follow-up (4-8 years).

　　　(**❶**　　　　　　　　　　　　　　　　　　　　　　　)を評価するため、
ALLHATは(**❷**　　　　　　　　　　　　　　　　　　　　　)と
(**❸**　　　　　　　　　　　　　　　　　　)でデザインされた。

2. <u>This study presents</u> results of the amlodipine and lisinopril <u>vs</u> chlorthalidone comparisons on major CVD outcomes.

　　　この試験は、(**❹**　　　　　　　　　　)を対照として、(**❺**　　　　　　　　　)
と(**❻**　　　　　　　　)の(**❼**　　　　　　　　　　　)に対する結果を示す。

✏ Exercise 2

以下にIntroductionのムーブに特徴的なHint Expressionが示されています。それぞれ、①背景ムーブ、②先行研究ムーブ、③ギャップムーブ、④本研究ムーブいずれのHint Expressionでしょうか？空所に該当する番号を書き入れましょう。

❶ Recently…has drawn much attention.　　　　　　　　　　(　　)
❷ Here, we evaluated whether…　　　　　　　　　　　　　(　　)
❸ As Kosugi et al. showed in their previous research…　　　(　　)
❹ Agent A has been widely used for patients with…　　　　(　　)
❺ Although … has been extensively studied, there is no consensus on…　(　　)
❻ There are many commercially available devices …　　　　(　　)
❼ The present study was aimed at …　　　　　　　　　　　(　　)
❽ Generally, Drug A is used for…　　　　　　　　　　　　(　　)
❾ Recent clinical trials have demonstrated benefits for…　　(　　)
❿ This study aims to…　　　　　　　　　　　　　　　　　(　　)
⓫ Further research is necessary to clarify…　　　　　　　　(　　)
⓬ In this research, we explore…　　　　　　　　　　　　　(　　)
⓭ …has not been fully studied.　　　　　　　　　　　　　　(　　)

69

⒁ It was suggested in the preclinical research that… （　　　）

⒂ Despite the substantial needs, few agents are available … （　　　）

✐ Applying what you learned

Introduction以降の論文本文には、数行にわたる長い文が多く見受けられますが、それを日本語の語順に合わせて後ろから訳すと意味が分からなくなってしまいます。英語の論文を読解するときにはまず、意味上のかたまり（句や節）を考えながらスラッシュ（斜線）で区切り、それぞれが文の構造上どのような役割を果たしているか分析して意味を理解することが大切です。

A. 論文に記載される文の主語(S)は、長い名詞句で表現されている場合が多くあります。次の文にスラッシュを入れ、日本語訳の空欄を埋めて意味を確認しましょう。

Several newer classes of antihypertensive agents (ie*, angiotensin-converting enzyme [ACE] inhibitors, calcium channel blockers [CCBs], α-adrenergic blockers, and more recently angiotensin-receptor blockers) became available.

*ie: ラテン語のid estの略で、「すなわち、つまり、言い換えると」という意味を持ち、「アイイー」と発音します。

（■❶　　　　　　　　　　　　　　　　　　　　　）（すなわち、アンジオテンシン変換酵素[ACE]阻害薬、カルシウムチャネル遮断薬[CCBs]、α-アドレナリン遮断薬、そしてより最近ではアンジオテンシン受容体遮断薬）が（■❷　　　　　　　　　　　　　　　）

B. 次の長文では、主語にあたる部分 "The Antihypertensive and Lipid-Lowering Treatment to Prevent Heart Attack Trial (ALLHAT)"（＝A）が、コンマの後、別の表現（＝B）で言い換えられています。このような場合、「AとBは同格である」と言います。

また、to determine以下は、「～かどうかを検証するために」と研究が行われた目的が記されています。determineの目的語であるwhether以下は主語(S)と動詞(V)を含むもうひとつ文がある「入れ子構造」になっています。このような場合は、文の構造を考えながら、前から順番に意味を確認していくと文全体が理解しやすくなります。

最初に、文全体にスラッシュを入れましょう。

The Antihypertensive and Lipid-Lowering Treatment to Prevent Heart Attack Trial (ALLHAT), a randomized, double-blind, multicenter clinical trial sponsored by the National Heart, Lung, and Blood Institute, was designed to determine whether the occurrence of fatal CHD or nonfatal myocardial infarction is lower for high-risk patients with hypertension treated with a CCB (represented by amlodipine), an ACE inhibitor (represented by lisinopril), or an α-blocker (represented by doxazosin), each compared with diuretic treatment (represented by chlorthalidone).

次に、スラッシュで区切られた各部分がどのような役割をしているかを分析します。

まず、to determineより前の文の構造を考えながら解答欄に該当する英語を当てはめ、対応する日本語訳の空欄を埋めましょう。

主語A: The Antihypertensive and Lipid-Lowering Treatment to Prevent Heart Attack Trial (ALLHAT)

主語Aと同格のB: **3**

どこから資金提供された: **4**

動詞 (V): **5**

ALLHAT試験、すなわち、(**6**　　　　　　　　　　　　　　　　) から資金提供を受けた
(**7**　　　　　　　　　　　　　　　　　) はデザインされた

次にto determine〜lowerまでの文の主語にあたる部分と動詞を特定して解答欄に英語で記入し、日本語訳の空欄に埋めましょう。

To determine whether…:〜かどうかを検証するために

主語(S): **8**

動詞(V): **9**

(**10**　　　　　　　　　　　　　　　　　　　　　　　　　　)
かどうかを検証するために

71

残りの部分ではALLHAT試験の対象となった参加者と、投与された治療薬およびその比較対照
薬について記載されています。解答欄に英語で情報を整理し、日本語訳の空欄を埋めましょう。

ALLHATの参加者：⓫

treated with

治療薬　　⓬

　　　　　⓭　　　　　　　　　　　　　　　　　　　　　　　　　　　　or

　　　　　⓮

each compared with

比較対照薬　⓯

（⓰　　　　　　　　　　　　　　　　　　　　　　　　　　　）、

（⓱　　　　　　　　　　　　　　　　　　　　　　　　　　）または

（⓲　　　　　　　　　　　　　　　　　　　　　　　　　　）による

治療を受けた（⓳　　　　　　　　　　　　　　　　　　　）患者において、

それぞれ（⓴　　　　　　　　　　　　　　　　　）による治療と比較して

72　*Lesson 10*

Lesson *11*

Research Article 3: Methods
臨床試験の原著論文を読む（3）　研究方法

　Lesson 11では、この論文で報告されている研究が実際にどのような方法で実施されたのかを示すMethods（研究方法）ついて学びます。MethodsはMaterials and Methods, Experiments, Proceduresなど雑誌によって呼び名が異なります。

▶ Getting to know the genre

Genre: 原著論文の「研究方法」

- **Purpose:** 　　　　研究手法を示す
- **Audience:** 　　　　医療専門家、研究者
- **Information:** 　　　試験デザイン、研究対象、介入、評価項目、分析手法
- **Linguistic features:** 受動態、過去形、無生物主語

◎ Checking the terms

approval	承認	physician's discretion	医師の裁量
assess	評価する	post hoc	事後に
assign	割り付ける	prespecify	事前に定める
encapsulate	カプセルで包む	primary outcome	主要転帰
exclude	除外する	safety outcome	安全性転帰
goal BP (Blood Pressure)	目標血圧	secondary outcome	副次的転帰
history of	〜の既往歴	statistical method	統計方法
institutional review board（IRB）	施設内治験審査委員会		
measurement	測定、計測		

Reading the text

Lesson 11では、Exerciseで取り上げる箇所のみ原文を表示しています。以下のURLからALLHATの原著にアクセスして、Methods全体に目を通しましょう。

https://jamanetwork.com/journals/jama/fullarticle/195626

Exercise 1

Methods（研究方法）では、Introductionで提示された論点に応えるために何をしたかが記されます。この論文ではStudy Design、Treatment、Outcomes、Statistical Methodsの4つに区切られており、それぞれ①「誰/どのような対象に」②「何をして」③「どのようなデータを取り」④「どのように分析したか」というMethodsセクションのムーブに対応しています。

A. Study Design（試験デザイン/参加者情報）

　　Methodsの第一のムーブであるStudy Designを確認しましょう。

臨床試験の論文を読むときは、まずその試験の対象となった参加者を規定する適格性基準（eligibility criteria）を確認することが大切です。Eligibilityは選択基準（inclusion criteria）と除外基準（exclusion criteria）に分けられます。

1. 以下の文を読んで、ALLHATの対象となった参加者の選択基準と除外基準を日本語で表にまとめましょう。Hint Expression(HE)に下線が引かれているので参考にしましょう。

The rationale and design of ALLHAT have been presented elsewhere.[18] Participants were men and women aged 55 years or older who had stage 1 or stage 2 hypertension with at least 1 additional risk factor for CHD events.[18,22] The risk factors included previous (>6 months) myocardial infarction or stroke, left ventricular hypertrophy demonstrated by electrocardiography or echocardiography, history of type 2 diabetes, current cigarette smoking, high-density lipoprotein cholesterol of less than 35 mg/dL (<0.91 mmol/L), or documentation of other atherosclerotic CVD. Individuals with a history of hospitalized or treated symptomatic heart failure (HF) and/or* known left ventricular ejection fraction of less than 35% were excluded.

参加者情報「誰/どのような対象に」	
選択基準	・性別：**1** ・年齢：**2** ・高血圧ステージ1または2であり、更に一つ以上のCHDイベントのリスクファクターを持つ。リスクファクターには以下が含まれる： 　　**3** 　　**4** 　　**5** 　　**6** 　　**7** 　　**8**
除外基準	**9**

※Study Designの冒頭の一文は、ALLHAT試験の実施根拠とデザインの詳細が他の文献[文献番号18]に提示されているという意味です。論文の最後にあるReferences（参考文献）にリストされている文献番号18を確認しましょう。
*and/orの使い方についてはp.79を参照。

74 *Lesson 11*

2. 以下の文を読んで、試験デザインの情報を表にまとめましょう。HEには下線を引いているので参考にしましょう。

By telephone, <u>participants were randomly assigned to</u> chlorthalidone, amlodipine, or lisinopril <u>in a ratio of</u> 1.7:1:1. The concealed randomization scheme was generated by computer, implemented at the clinical trials center, stratified by center and blocked in random block sizes of 5 or 9 to maintain balance. <u>Participants (n = 33 357) were recruited at</u> 623 centers in the
5 United States, Canada, Puerto Rico, and the US Virgin Islands between February 1994 and January 1998. (The original reported number of 625 sites changed because 2 sites and their patients with poor documentation of informed consent were excluded.[20] All participants gave written informed consent, and all centers obtained institutional review board approval**. <u>Follow-up visits were at</u> 1 month; 3, 6, 9, and 12 months; and every 4 months thereafter. <u>The</u>
10 <u>range of possible follow-up was</u> 3 years 8 months to 8 years 1 month. The closeout phase began on October 1, 2001 and ended on March 31, 2002.

試験デザイン			
治験薬割付比率	クロルサリドン ＝ 🔟	：アムロジピン ：⑪	：リシノプリル ：⑫
参加者と施設情報	⑬総参加者数： ⑭参加施設数： ⑮参加施設の所在地： ⑯参加者募集期間：		
参加者の施設訪問日	⑰		
追跡期間	⑱	〜⑲	

**All participants gave written informed consent, and all centers obtained institutional review board approval（全参加者は文書で試験参加に同意し、全ての参加施設は施設治験審査委員会の承認を得た）という文は、臨床試験の論文ではmethodsに記述される定型的な文です。

B. Treatment（治療）

   Treatmentのムーブでは、この臨床試験でどのような治療を行ったのか、その内容や薬剤の投与計画などが詳細に述べられます。

   下線部のHEを参考にしながら、この臨床試験の治療内容を表にまとめましょう。

Trained observers using standardized techniques measured BPs during the trial.[20] Visit BP was the average of 2 seated measurements. Goal BP in each randomized group was <u>less than</u> 140/90 mm Hg achieved by titrating the <u>assigned study drug</u> (step 1) and adding <u>open-label</u> <u>agents</u> (step 2 or 3) when necessary. The choice of step 2 drugs (atenolol, clonidine, or
5 reserpine) was <u>at the physician's discretion</u>. Nonpharmacologic approaches to treatment of hypertension were recommended according to national guidelines.[4,23] Step 1 drugs were

75

encapsulated and identical in appearance so that the identity of each agent was double-masked* at each dosage level. Dosages were 12.5, 12.5 (sham titration**), and 25 mg/d for chlorthalidone; 2.5, 5, and 10 mg/d for amlodipine; and 10, 20, and 40 mg/d for lisinopril. Doses of study-supplied open-label step 2 drugs were 25 to 100 mg/d of atenolol; 0.05 to 0.2 mg/d of reserpine; or 0.1 to 0.3 mg twice a day of clonidine; step 3 was 25 to 100 mg twice a day of hydralazine. Other drugs, including low doses of open-label step 1 drug classes, were permitted if clinically indicated.[18,20]

* double-masked：double-blindと同義で、研究者、参加者ともに割り付けられた薬剤を知らないという意味
** sham titration：偽の漸増（盲検下で増量しているつもりが実際は同じ用量を継続している）

治療「何をしたか」				
・目標血圧は、収縮期(最高)血圧 (**1**) mmHg/拡張期(最小)血圧：(**2**) mmHg (**3**)で、(**4**)(step 1)の用量を漸増しながら達成し (**5**)(step 2 or 3)を必要に応じて追加した。				
・ステップ2の薬剤(アテノロール、クロニジンまたはレセルピン)の選択は (**6**)で行った。				
・ステップ1の薬剤は、それぞれの薬剤の各用量レベルで外見が二重にマスクされるよう (**7**)				
ステップ1薬の 漸増計画	クロルサリドン：**8** アムロジピン ：**11** リシノプリル ：**14**	mg/日→**9** mg/日→**12** mg/日→**15**	mg/日→**10** mg/日→**13** mg/日→**16**	mg/日 mg/日 mg/日
ステップ2薬の用量	アテノロール ：**17** レセルピン ：**19** クロニジン ：**21**	～**18** ～**20** ～**22**	mg/日 mg/日 mg 1日**23**	回
ステップ3薬の用量	ヒドララジン ：**24**	～ **25**	mg/日 1日**26**	回

76 *Lesson 11*

C. Outcomes（転帰）

Outcomesのムーブでは、この臨床試験でどのようなデータをとって治療の効果を比較したのか、その評価項目が示されています。

1. この臨床試験の主要転帰（primary outcome）と副次的転帰（secondary outcome）を日本語で表にまとめましょう。

The primary outcome was fatal CHD or nonfatal myocardial infarction combined.[18] Four major prespecified* secondary outcomes were all-cause mortality, fatal and nonfatal stroke, combined CHD (the primary outcome, coronary revascularization, hospitalized angina), and combined CVD (combined CHD, stroke, other treated angina, HF [fatal, hospitalized, or treated nonhospitalized], and peripheral arterial disease).

転帰（評価項目）「どのようなデータを取ったか」	
Primary outcome 主要転帰	**1**
Four major prespecified secondary outcomes 4つの主な副次的転帰	・**2** ・**3** ・combined CHD（複合CHD） 　　　**4** 　　　**5** 　　　**6** ・combined CVD（複合CVD） 　　　**7** 　　　**8** 　　　**9** 　　　**10** 　　　**11**

2. この臨床試験の安全性転帰（safety outcome）を日本語でまとめましょう。

Two major safety outcomes, angioedema and hospitalization for gastrointestinal bleeding, were prespecified*.

Two major safety outcomes 2つの主な安全性転帰	**12** **13**

*prespecified（事前に定めた）とは、臨床試験が始まる前に評価項目を規定することを指し、これに対して臨床試験の開始後に追加した評価項目はpost-hoc（事後に）で表す。

77

D. Statistical Methods

統計手法（statistical methods）のムーブでは、臨床試験から得られたデータをどのように分析するかが記述されています。下表の統計解析に関連する用語を参考にして本文を読みましょう。

統計手法「どのように分析したか」			
statistical power	検出力	cumulative event rate	累積イベント発生率
sample size	サンプルサイズ（被験者数）	Kaplan-Meier method	カプランマイヤー法
expected event rate	推定イベント発生率	log-rank test	ログランク検定
treatment crossover	治療クロスオーバー	cox proportional hazards regression model	コックス比例ハザード回帰モデル
losses to follow-up	追跡不能（者数）	hazard ratio (relative risk [RR])	ハザード比（相対危険度[RR]）
2-sided	両側の	95% confidence interval (CIs)	95%信頼区間（CI）
intent-to-treat analysis	ITT解析	2-by-2 table	2 x 2表

統計手法ムーブのHint Expression（下線部）を確認しながら以下の文を日本語にしましょう。

1. x times as many A as B（AはBのx倍）

この表現について注意すべき点は、A と B が文法的に等価であることです。次の文では、論文本文では重複を避けるために省略されている語を括弧内に補っています。

To maximize statistical power, 1.7 <u>times as many</u> participants were assigned to the diuretic group <u>as</u> (participants were assigned) to each of the other 3 groups.

検出力を（**1**   ）、利尿薬群にはその他の3つの治療群
の（**2**   ）

2. 前提条件を表すgiven

given…は前提条件を表す表現で、「…を前提とすると」「…であると仮定すると」といった日本語で表現することができます。以下の文では、83%という検出力が得られた計算式に入力した数値の項目が述べられています。

<u>Given the achieved sample size and expected event rate, treatment crossovers, and losses to follow-up</u>, ALLHAT had 83% power to detect a 16% reduction in risk of the primary outcome between chlorthalidone and each other group

（**3**   ）
を前提とすると、ALLHAT試験は、クロルサリドン群と他の各治療群間の16%の主要転帰リスク低

下を検出する83%の検出力を持っていた。

✏➤ Exercise 2

Methodsに記されている重要な文法事項やよく使われる表現を見ておきましょう。

A. 数字の「以上・以下」、「超・未満」の表現

以上	…or more, …or aboveなど	超*	more than, over, aboveなど
以下	…or less, …or belowなど	未満	less than, under, belowなど

*その数字を含まない、その数字を超えて

以下の文の（　　）内に、以上、以下、超、未満のいずれかを入れましょう。

1. Participants were men and women aged 55 years or older.
   参加者は55歳（**1**　　　）の男女であった。

2. The risk factors included high-density lipoprotein cholesterol of less than 35 mg/dL.
   リスクファクターはHDLコレステロール35 mg/dL（**2**　　　）を含んだ。

3. Goal BP in each randomized group was less than 140/90 mmHg.
   各割り付け群の血圧目標は140/90 mmHg（**3**　　　）であった。

B. 特殊な接続表現　A and/or B
"A and/or B"という表現は、"A and B" or "A or B"、すなわち「AとBの両方、または、AかBのいずれか」という意味を持ちます。

Individuals with a history of hospitalized or treated symptomatic heart failure (HF) and/or known left ventricular ejection fraction of less than 35% were excluded.

上の文でAとBに当たる部分にアンダーラインを引き、文の意味を確認しましょう。
試験から除外された患者は、① individuals with A, ② individuals with B, ③ individuals with A and B ということになります。

C. 括弧の種類と使用
括弧で情報をくくる場合は、まず丸括弧（　）を用い、（　）の中の情報を更にくくる場合は角括弧[　]を用います。
Four major prespecified secondary outcomes were all-cause mortality, fatal and nonfatal stroke, combined CHD (the primary outcome, coronary revascularization, hospitalized angina), and combined CVD (combined CHD, stroke, other treated angina, HF [fatal, hospitalized, or treated nonhospitalized], and peripheral arterial disease).

79

Lesson 12

Research Article 4: Results
臨床試験の原著論文を読む（4）　結果

　Lesson 12ではResults（結果）を学習します。Resultsでは、臨床試験から得られた詳細な結果がデータとともに報告されます。このセクションを読む際には、詳細な結果報告から、いかにして重要な情報を効率的に得るかがポイントとなります。

Getting to know the genre

Genre: 原著論文の「結果」

- **Purpose:** Methods に記された研究方法に従って得た結果を客観的に提示する
- **Audience:** 医療専門家、研究者
- **Information:** 事実（著者の考えは含まない）、数値データを示す図表
- **Linguistic features:** 無生物主語や受動態、定量的な表現 、動詞は過去形

Checking the terms

adherence	遵守
baseline	ベースライン（測定の基線）
consistent	一致する、一貫性がある
decrease	減少する
distribution	分布
ESRD (End-Stage Renal Disease)	末期の腎疾患
figure	図
observed	観察された

overall	全体の
peripheral arterial disease	末梢動脈疾患
respectively	それぞれ
seated BP	座って測った血圧
significant	（統計学的に）有意な
stroke	脳卒中
table	表

Reading the text

Lesson 12では、Exerciseで取り上げる箇所のみ原文を表示しています。以下のURLからALLHATの原著にアクセスして、Results全体に目を通しましょう。

https://jamanetwork.com/journals/jama/fullarticle/195626

Exercise 1

Resultsでは、試験結果を図表を参照しながら報告します。著者の主観的な考察は含まず、得られた結果が客観的に記述され、①無生物主語や受動態、②定量的な表現（differ, increase, decreaseなどの動詞、higher, lowerなど形容詞の比較級）③動詞の時制は主に過去形を使用する*ことなどが特徴です。Resultsはいくつかのサブセクションに分けられていますが、ここでは最も重要なサブセクションであるPrimary and Secondary Outcomesを読みましょう。Methodsの転帰（outcomes）のムーブに記されているPrimary Outcome（主要転帰）とSecondary Outcomes（副次的転帰）の項目に従って結果が報告されていることに注目しましょう。Primary and Secondary Outcomesは更に、2群間の比較ごとに2つの下位サブセクションに分けられています。

*図表の説明では論文そのものに視点があるため、"Table 1 presents"や"Figures 1 shows"など現在形で書かれています。

A. Amlodipine vs Chlorthalidone

以下の文の構造を考えながら文中にスラッシュ（斜線）を入れて分解し、解答欄に英語のまま書き込みましょう。次に、対応する日本語訳の空欄に適切な言葉を埋めながら内容を理解しましょう。

Hint Expressions (HE)には線が引いてあります。

1. No significant difference was observed between amlodipine and chlorthalidone for the primary outcome or for the secondary outcomes of all-cause mortality, combined CHD, stroke, combined CVD, angina, coronary revascularization, peripheral arterial disease, cancer, or ESRD (Table 5, Figure 3, and Figure 4).

主語：**1**　　　　　　　　　　　　　　動詞：**2**
何と何の比較で：**3**
何について1：**4**

                              or

何について2：**5**

（**6**　　　　　　　　　　　）群と（**7**　　　　　　　　　　　）群の間で（**8**　　　　　　　　　）な
差は観察されなかった
　　（**9**　　　　　　　　　　）について、あるいは
　　（**10**　　　　　　　　　　）の以下の項目について
　　　　（**11**　　　　　　　　）（**12**　　　　　　　　）（**13**　　　　　　　）（**14**　　　　　　　）
　　　　（**15**　　　　　　　　）（**16**　　　　　　　　）（**17**　　　　　　　）（**18**　　　　　　　）
　　　　（**19**　　　　　　　　）
参照すべき図表：表（**20**　　　　　　　）
　　　　　　　　　図（**21**　　　　　　　）

2. The amlodipine group had a 38% higher risk of HF (P <.001) with a 6-year absolute risk difference of 2.5% and a 35% higher risk of hospitalized/fatal HF (P <.001).

```
主語: 22                          動詞: 23
目的語1: 24
補足事項: 25
                                  and
目的語2: 26
```

アムロジピン群は（クロルサリドン群と比較して）、
(27   ) (P <.001)、
（補足事項: 28   ）
また、(29   ) (P <.001)。

B. Lisinopril vs Chlorthalidone

　以下の文1と2は、上記**A.1.**および**A.2.**で紹介した文とほぼ同じ構造をしていることがわかります。空欄を適切な言葉で埋めましょう。

1. No significant difference was observed between lisinopril and chlorthalidone for the primary outcome (RR, 0.99; 95% CI, 0.91-1.08) or for the secondary outcomes of all-cause mortality, combined CHD, peripheral arterial disease, cancer, or ESRD (Table 5, Figure 3 and Figure 4).

(**1**   ) (RR, 0.99; 95% CI, 0.91-1.08)、あるいは(**2**   )の
(**3**   )の各項目について、(**4**   )
の間に(**5**   )

参照すべき図表: 表(**6**   ) 図(**7**   )

2. The lisinopril group had a 15% higher risk for stroke (P = .02) and a 10% higher risk of combined CVD (P<.001), with a 6-year absolute risk difference for combined CVD of 2.4%.

リシノプリル群は（クロルサリドン群と比較して）、
　　(**8**   ) (P = .02)、
また、(**9**   ) (P <.001)、
複合CVDの6年の絶対リスク差は2.4%であった。

3. Included in this analysis was [sic] a 19% higher risk of HF (P<.001), a 10% higher risk of hospitalized/fatal HF (P = .11), an 11% higher risk of hospitalized/treated angina (P = .01), and a 10% higher risk of coronary revascularization (P = .05).

この文は、文頭にoutcomesという語を補うとわかりやすいです。

```
主語：Outcomes ❿                     動詞：⓫
補語1： ⓬
補語2： ⓭
補語3： ⓮
and
補語4： ⓯
```

（⓰   ）には、
（⓱   ）(P<.001)、
（⓲   ）(P = .11)、
（⓳   ）(P = .01)、そして
（⓴   ）(P = .05)があった。

C. Table 5

上記Primary and Secondary Outocomesの2つのサブセクションの内容をTable 5で確認しましょう。

Table 5. Clinical Outcomes by Antihypertensive Treatment Group

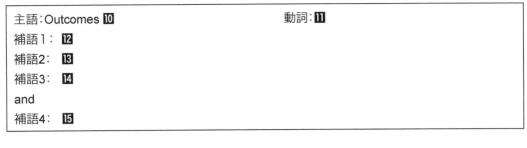

1. **A.** Amlodipine vs Chlorthalidoneの記述に対応する転帰項目と関連するP値*について、Table 5の該当箇所に印を付けましょう。

2. **B.** Lisinopril vs Chlorthalidoneの記述に対応する転帰項目と関連するP値*について、Table 5の該当箇所に印を付けましょう。

*P値は「偶然性による影響で違いが出た」確率を示し、その値が小さいほど、違いが偶然生じたとは考えにくいということになります。従って、この値がじゅうぶんに小さければ、その項目については治療薬群間に、偶然ではない意味のある「有意差」があったと判定します。(値は、研究者が求める有意性の確実度によって異なりますが、一般的には＜0.05、高い確実度を求める場合は＜0.01などが採用されます。)

Exercise 2

Resultsに含まれる以下の文について、下線部のHEに注意しながら日本語に訳しましょう。また、音声を聞いて、数字や単位の読み方も練習しましょう。　　　　　　　(◀))Track12-1)

1 <u>Table 1 presents</u> baseline characteristics for the 33,357 participants in the chlorthalidone, amlodipine, and lisinopril treatment groups.

2 <u>There were nearly identical distributions of</u> baseline factors in the 3 treatment groups

3 <u>Figure 1 shows</u> the number of participants randomized and followed up to the time of close out.

4 <u>Mean</u> seated BP at randomization was about 146/84 mm Hg in all 3 group.

5 Visit adherence <u>decreased over time from</u> about 92% at 1 year <u>to</u> 84% <u>to</u> 87% at 5 years in all 3 treatment groups

6 Among participants with available medication information at 1 year, 26.7%, 25.9%, and 32.6% of those assigned to chlorthalidone, amlodipine, and lisinopril, <u>respectively</u>, were taking a step 2 or step 3 drug.

7 The treatment effects for all outcomes <u>were consistent across</u> subgroups by sex, diabetic status, and baseline CHD status.

8 <u>Significant differences were seen for</u> the lisinopril vs chlorthalidone comparison overall.

84 *Lesson 12*

Exercise 3

臨床試験の論文を読む際には、Results冒頭のPatient CharacteristicsとVisit and Medication Adherenceに含まれる情報を、それぞれ対応する図表と合わせて確認しておくことが重要です。

A. Patient Characteristics

Table 1	Baseline Characteristics of the ALLHAT Participants ALLHAT参加者のベースラインの背景因子と臨床特性

臨床試験で比較する治療薬の効果を正確に理解するためには、さまざまな偏り（バイアス）をできる限り排除する必要があります。比較する治療薬群間で参加者の背景因子や臨床特性に偏りがないことは、治療薬の効果を客観的に判定するための前提条件です。

1. どのような背景因子や臨床特性が記載されているか確認しましょう。
2. 多くの項目について3つの治療薬群間の数値が近似していて、治療薬群間の偏りが小さいことを確認しましょう。

B. Visit and Medication Adherence

Figure 1	Randomization and Follow-up of Participants in the Antihypertensive and Lipid-Lowering Treatment to Prevent Heart Attack Trial ALLHAT参加者の無作為化と追跡期間中の経過
Table 2	Visits Expected and Completed and Antihypertensive Medication Use at Annual Visits 各年の訪問日の予定来院者数と実際の来院者数および高血圧治療薬の使用状況

Figure 1では、割付け後に各群の参加者がどの時点で何人脱落したか、試験終了時点の参加者の状況、この試験の解析対象となった人数が記載されています。無作為化試験の論文ではFigure 1にあたる図がほとんどの場合示されており、統計解析の対象となった集団が確認できます。ITT解析の場合は試験開始時に各群に割付けられた人数と最終的に解析対象として含まれた人数が一致していることがわかります。

またTable 2では、各群の参加者の来院状況や、服薬遵守状況を把握することができます。

1. 2984ページの "Visit adherence decreased over time from about 92% at 1 year to 84% to 87% at 5 years in all 3 treatment groups (Table 2)." をTable 2で確認しましょう。

85

Lesson *13*

Research Article 5: Discussion, Comment
臨床試験の原著論文を読む(5)　考察

　Lesson 13では、考察にあたるCommentを学習します。多くの論文で「考察」は Discussionと呼ばれます。Introduction（序論）では、その領域の研究がどのように社会と関連していていかに重要であるかという広い範囲から次第に論文の論点へと絞り込まれました。論文の最後のセクションであるCommentでは、著者が結果を解釈し、論点に対する解答を与えて結論へと導きます。研究から得られた知見が、Introductionで示した研究領域の中でどのように位置づけられ、臨床医学の発展や実地医療の進歩にとってどのように意義深い貢献であるかを読者に納得してもらうための重要なセクションです。

Getting to know the genre

Genre: 原著論文の「考察」

- **Purpose:**　　　　　　　研究から得られた知見の意義を読者に納得させる
- **Audience:**　　　　　　　医療専門家、研究者
- **Information:**　　　　　　結果の要約と解釈、先行研究との比較、研究の限界、将来の展望、
　　　　　　　　　　　　　　得られた知見の適用範囲、結論
- **Linguistic features:**　　動詞の時制の使い分け、助動詞の適切な使用

Checking the terms

be blinded	が分からない	release	発売する
consistent with	〜に一致する	survival	生存
evaluate	評価する	tolerability	忍容性
finding	結果、知見	unsurpassed	超えられない
indicate	示す、示唆する	urge	奨励する
limitation	限界	worth noting	言及（注目）に値する
reinforce	強固にする		

Reading the text

Lesson 13では、Exerciseで取り上げる箇所のみ原文を表示しています。以下のURLから ALLHATの原著にアクセスして、Comment全体に目を通しましょう。

https://jamanetwork.com/journals/jama/fullarticle/195626

86　*Lesson 13*

Exercise 1

Commentは、通常、①Introductionで示された論点に対する解答と考察、②研究の限界、③結論という流れ（ムーブ）で書かれています。事実としての結果を客観的に記述するResultsとは対照的に、主観を表す動詞や助動詞が多く使われることが特徴です。

A. 結果の考察
結果の考察ムーブは、論点に対する解答から始まり、先行研究と対比させながら結果の正当性を裏付けます。

1. 次の文は、Commentの最初の文です。'Neither A nor B…'（AもBも…ではない）の構文に注意して、対応する日本語訳の空欄に適切な言葉を埋めましょう。Hint Expressions (HE)に下線が引いてあります。

<u>Neither</u> amlodipine (representing CCBs, particularly dihydropyridine [DHP]–CCBs) <u>nor</u> lisinopril (representing ACE inhibitors) <u>was superior to</u> chlorthalidone (representing thiazide-type diuretics) <u>in preventing</u> major coronary events <u>or in increasing</u> survival.

アムロジピン（**1**　　　　　　　　を代表する）も、リシノプリル（**2**　　　　　　　　を代表する）も、（**3**　　　　　　　）の予防、あるいは（**4**　　　　　　　　）の増加という点で、クロルサリドン（**5**　　　　　　　　を代表する）に（**6**　　　　　　　　）。

2. 先行研究と一致する点だけでなく矛盾する点についても言及します。下線部のHint Expressions (HE) に注目して、対応する日本語訳の空欄に適切な言葉を埋めましょう。

・The amlodipine vs chlorthalidone findings for HF <u>reinforce previous trial results</u>.
心不全に対するアムロジピンとクロルサリドンの比較から得た知見は、（**7**　　　　　　　　）。

・<u>The ALLHAT findings</u> for some major outcomes <u>are consistent with</u> predictions from placebo-controlled trials involving ACE inhibitors and diuretics.

一部の主要な転帰に対するALLHAT試験から得た知見は、ACE阻害薬と利尿薬を投与した（**8**　　　）試験からの予測と（**9**　　　　　　　）。

・<u>The results of ALLHAT do not support these findings</u>. <u>In fact</u>, the mortality from noncardiovascular causes <u>was significantly lower</u> in the CCB group.

ALLHAT試験の結果はこれらの知見を（**10**　　　　　　　　）。実際、非心臓血管系の原因による死亡率はCCB群において（**11**　　　　　　　）。

87

B. 研究の限界

結果の限界ムーブでは、研究の限界（limitation）について述べる他、その研究の範囲外の事項や将来検討されるべき課題が記述されます。下線部のHEに注目して文を観察しましょう。

・<u>Some limitations are worth noting</u>. After ALLHAT was designed, newer agents have been or may soon be released (eg, angiotensin-receptor blockers, selective aldosterone antagonists), <u>which were not evaluated</u>.

（**1**   ）。ALLHAT試験がデザインされた後で、より新しい薬剤（例えば、アンジオテンシン受容体ブロッカー、選択的アルドステロン拮抗薬）が発売された、あるいは間もなく発売される可能性があり、それらは（**2**   ）。

・<u>Although</u> clinical centers were <u>blinded to</u> the regimen and urged to achieve recommended BP goals, equivalent BP reduction <u>was not fully achieved</u> in the treatment groups.

臨床センター（試験施設）は治療計画について（**3**   ）、推奨血圧目標を達成するよう奨励されていたが、治療薬群において、同等の血圧低下は（**4**   ）。

C. 結論

論文の最後は結論（conclusion）で締めくくられます。結論は考察と独立して書かれる場合もあります。臨床試験の結論では、判断や思考など主観を表す助動詞（例：should）や動詞（例：consider）を使い、研究結果を踏まえて臨床現場ではどうすればよいかを示唆します。また、動詞は現在形が用いられます。

結論部分の第1文を下線部のHEに注目しながら日本語に訳しましょう。

・<u>In conclusion</u>, the results of ALLHAT indicate that thiazide-type diuretics <u>should be considered first for</u> pharmacologic therapy <u>in patients with</u> hypertension. <u>They are unsurpassed in</u> lowering BP, reducing clinical events, and tolerability, <u>and they are</u> less costly.

結論として、ALLHAT試験の結果は、高血圧患者における薬物療法として、サイアザイド系利尿薬を（**1**   ）。それら（＝**2**   ）は、（**3**   ）において優るものはなく、またそれらは費用もより安価である。

Applying what you learned

興味があるテーマの論文をPubMedで検索して、ダウンロードしてください。授業で習った読み方を参考に内容を理解し、概要をクラスに紹介してみましょう。

・論文情報：タイトル　ジャーナル名　著者名　掲載年
・序論：背景と研究目的
・研究方法：①研究対象/被験者　②介入/治療（薬剤投与デザインなど）　③評価項目（転帰など）
・結果と結論：評価項目における結果と関連する図表、結論

Appendix

1 イギリス英語・アメリカ英語の違い

A. Spelling（綴り）・表現

本書に出てくる表現は太字で示しています。

Lesson	イギリス英語	アメリカ英語	日本語訳
L1, L2	**diarrhoea** (L2)	diarrhea (L1)	下痢
L2	**casualty department***	emergency room (ER)	救急救命部
L2	**discolouration**	discoloration	変色
L2, L6	**hyperglycaemia**	hyperglycemia	低血糖
L2	**paediatric**	pediatric	小児の
L2	**haemodynamically**	hemodynamically	血行動態的に
L2	**oedema**	edema	浮腫
L2	**hyperkalaemia**	hyperkalemia	高カリウム血症
L3	**foetus**	fetus	胎児
L4	**fibre**	fiber	繊維
L4, L6	**surgery**** (L4)	**clinic**** (L6)	診療所
L6, L7	counselling	**counseling**	カウンセリング
L7	**dyslipidaemia**	dyslipidemia	脂質異常症
L7	antidyslipidaemic	**antidyslipidemic**	脂質異常症治療薬・抗脂質異常症薬
L7	tranquiliser	**tranquilizer**	鎮静薬
L8	neutralised/neutralisation	**neutralized/ neutralization**	中和された/中和
L9-L13	randomised	**randomized**	無作為化
L9-L13	centre	**center**	センター/中心
L9-L13	revascularisation	**revascularization**	血管再建/再灌流
L9-L13	hospitalisation	**hospitalization**	入院

*casualty departmentはaccident and emergency (A&E) departmentともいう（イギリス）。
**アメリカでsurgeryは「手術」という意味のみ。clinic「診療所」はイギリスでも使われる。

B. その他の違い

1. 英米で同じ綴りの単語でも発音が異なるものもあるので注意しましょう。例えばvitaminの最初のiの発音はイギリスでは短いイ [vɪtəmɪn] ですが、アメリカではアイ [vaɪtəmɪn] です。

2. Mr. Ms. Dr. などアメリカ英語の略字の後にはピリオドが使われますが、イギリス英語ではピリオドを使わずMr Ms Drとなります。

3. 英米では使用する単位が異なる場合があります。イギリスでは一般的にも摂氏・メートル法が用いられますが、アメリカでは温度は華氏、身長や体重はfeet, poundが用いられます。

90

2 おすすめの無料サイト

A. 無料辞書・用語解説

1. 英辞郎 on the WEB: http://www.alc.co.jp/
   ALCが提供している英和・和英対訳データベース。専門用語も広くカバーしている。

2. Weblio: https://ejje.weblio.jp/
   英和・和英辞書だけではなく、類語辞書もある日本最大級の辞書サイト。発音も聞くことができ、用例も豊富で例文検索もできる。

3. Howjsay: http://www.howjsay.com
   音声で数多くの専門用語の発音を確認できるサイト。英米の発音が異なる場合はそれぞれ確認できる。

4. 医学英語語幹：http://www.medo.jp/a.htm
   日本人医師が制作、提供している語幹と接頭・接尾辞のサイト。

5. Life Science Dictionary：https://lsd-project.jp/cgi-bin/lsdproj/ejlookup04.pl
   生命科学（ライフサイエンス）領域で使われる専門用語、対訳、用法のサイト。

6. OneLook dictionary search：https://www.onelook.com/
   英語母語話者用だが、主要な英英辞典を1か所で検索できる。

7. 英語非母語話者用の英英辞書：
   平易な英語で説明しているので、患者に説明する言い換えの表現の参考として使える。
   ● Cambridge Learner's Dictionary*: https://dictionary.cambridge.org/ja/dictionary/learner-english/
   ● Oxford Learner's Dictionaries*: https://www.oxfordlearnersdictionaries.com/
   ● Merriam-Webster's Learner's Dictionary: http://www.learnersdictionary.com/
   *ケンブリッジとオックスフォードはイギリス英語とアメリカ英語の発音付き

8. 薬学用語解説：https://www.pharm.or.jp/dictionary/wiki.cgi
   社団法人日本薬学会が編集した用語解説サイト。日本語での解説だが、英語の用語も掲載されている。

B. 学習サイト

MediEigo: http://medieigo.com/
医療現場で使える英語フレーズ集を始め、医学論文頻出語や医療系のニュースなど内容が充実している学習サイト。

3 薬局や病院での英語

A. 服薬指導に役立つ表現集

1. 服用回数

1日1回	once a day, once daily
1日2回	twice a day, two times daily
1日3回	three times a day, three times daily

2. 服用時間・タイミング

朝食後	after breakfast	食間 (空腹時)	between meals (on your empty stomach)
昼食後	after lunch	起床時	right after waking up
夕食後	after dinner	就寝前	at bedtime, before going to sleep /bed
毎食後	after every meal after meals	必要時、頓服	when necessary as needed
毎食前	before meals	__ 時間ごと	every __ hours
毎食直後	right/immediately after meals	少なくとも__時間以上あける	leave at least __ hours apart leave at least __ hours between doses
毎食直前	right/immediately before meals	隔日	every other day on alternate days

3. 医薬品の剤型

錠剤	tablet	点鼻スプレー	nasal spray
カプセル	capsule	吸入剤	inhaler
散剤	powder	軟膏	ointment
顆粒/細粒	granule/fine granule	点眼液	eye drops
注射薬	injection	湿布	patch
舌下錠	sublingual tablet	貼付薬	patch
チュアブル錠	chewable tablet	坐薬	suppository
OD錠	orally disintegrating tablet	トローチ	lozenge
包	packet, sachet	シロップ	syrup

4. 投与経路*

日本語	略語	英語	日本語	略語	英語
経口	PO, p.o.	per os, per oral	皮下	SC, s.c.	subcutaneous
経鼻胃	NG	nasogastric	筋肉内	IM	intramuscular
腹腔内	IP, i.p.	intraperitoneal	静脈内	IV, i.v.	intravenous
皮内	ID	intradermal	点滴静脈内	DIV	drip intravenous

*これらは専門的な表現で、日本でもカルテなどに略語が用いられます。一般の人には理解できないかもしれません。

B. 薬効別医薬品分類

日本語	専門的な表現	一般に用いられる表現
抗不整脈薬	antiarrhythmic	antiarrhythmic, medicine for heart beat
利尿薬	diuretic	water pill, water tablet
降圧薬	antihypertensive	high blood pressure reducer
抗血栓薬	antithrombotic	blood thinner
抗血小板薬	antiplatelet	
抗凝固薬	anticoagulant	
血糖降下剤	hypoglycemic agent/drug	blood sugar lowering agent/drug
脂質異常症治療薬	antidyslipidaemic[英], antidyslipidemic[米]	cholesterol reducer, cholesterol lowering agent/drug
鎮静薬	sedative, tranquiliser[英], tranquilizer[米]	nerve pill, nerve tablet, tranquiliser[英], tranquilizer[米]
抗不安薬	antianxiety agent/drug, antiolytic	antianxiety agent/drug
抗うつ薬	antidepressant	antidepressant
睡眠薬	hypnotic	sleeping pill
経口避妊薬	oral contraceptive	the pill
抗炎症薬	anti-inflammatory drug	anti-inflammatory drug
鎮痛薬	analgesic	painkiller
解熱薬	antipyretic	fever reliever
緩下薬	laxative	stool softener
制酸薬	antacid	antacid
抗ヒスタミン薬	antihistamine	allergy medicine
鎮咳薬	antitussive	cough medicine

C. ドラッグストアでよく見る商品カテゴリーと関連する表現

商品カテゴリー	関連する表現
Allergy, Asthma and Sinus	nasal spray, non-drowsy
Cough Cold and Flu	cough syrup, throat lozenge
Pain Relief	painkiller, migraine, menstrual, oral
Digestive Health	antacid, anti-diarrheal, gas relief, laxative
Skin Care	moisturizer, sun care, insect repellent
Oral Care	toothbrush, toothpaste, floss
Hair Care	shampoo, conditioner, scalp
Feminine Care	tampon, pad[米], liner, sanitary towel[英]
Baby Care	diaper[米], nappy[英], wipe, formula
Beauty	makeup product, nail
Diet and Nutrition	vitamin, supplement, herb
First Aid Supply	antiseptic, antibiotic, bandage

4 英語文書・資料作成の基本

英語で発表のスライドを作る時に参考にしてください。以下のサイトも参照しましょう。
https://www.thepunctuationguide.com/

A. Punctuation: コンピュータ上での英語表記の注意事項
　英語の入力法は日本語とかなり異なるので、慣れるまで意識して気を付けてください。コンピュータ上で間違いの箇所に波下線が表示されることもありますが、最後に必ず文書校正を行いましょう。

1. フォントの種類とサイズ
日本語は、全角入力しますが、英語では必ず半角で入力しましょう。そして、代表的な英語フォントの中から一つ選んで使用するようにしましょう。（よく使われる英語フォント例：Arial, Times New Roman, Microsoft San Serif, Comic Sans MS)

2. 言語
綴りや単語の選択はアメリカ英語もしくはイギリス英語に統一させましょう（P90 Appedix 1参照）。

3. スペースの空け方
半角スペースを空ける・空けないの区別は日本人にとっては非常に難しいですが、英語母語話者にはしっかりとした使い分けがあるので、気を付けましょう。

a. 半角スペースを1つあける場合
（1）ピリオド(.)の後　（2つでもよい。一貫性を持たせること）

（2）コンマの後
　　○ The patient had <u>diabetes, high blood pressure, and</u> cardiovascular disease.
　　× The patient had <u>diabetes,high blood pressure,and</u> cardiovascular disease.

（3）省略記号として用いられたピリオドの後
　　○ <u>Dr. R.</u> Jones left his office at 2:30 p.m.
　　× <u>Dr.R.</u> Jones left his office at 2:30 p.m.

（4）&の前後
　　○ Questions & Answers[*]　　Food & Beverages　　FDA & Regulatory Policy
　　× Questions&Answers[*]　　Food&Beverages　　FDA&Regulatory Policy
　　　[*]Q&Aと一つの単語のように見なされると&の前後のスペースは必要ない。

（5）括弧の外側　（内側にはあけない）

○ Shibasaburo Kitasato (1853-1931) was a famous bacteriologist.

× Shibasaburo Kitasato(1853-1931)was a famous bacteriologist.

× Shibasaburo Kitasato (1853-1931) was a famous bacteriologist.

(6) 引用符("") の外側（内側にはあけない）

○ The patient said, "I feel the pain right here."

× The patient said,"I feel the pain right here."

× The patient said, " I feel the pain right here. "

(7) 数学記号の前後

○ a + b = c   19.8 ± 1.5   n = 251

× a+b=c   19.8±1.5   n=251

(8) 数字と単位の間

○ 4.5 ml   6.0 km   2 mm Hg   10 mg/d

× 4.5ml   6.0km   2mmHg   10mg/d

b. スペースをあけてはいけない場合

(1) ハイフンとエヌダッシュの前後

語をつなぐ記号には2種類あり、ハイフン（-）よりエヌダッシュ（–）の方が長い。いずれの場合もスペースに関するルールは同じである。

○ 30–50 years old[*]   0.89–1.02   3-hydroxy-3-methylglutaryl coenzyme A

× 30 – 50 years old   0.89 – 1.02   3 - hydroxy - 3 - methylglutaryl coenzyme A

[*]日本語の「～」は用いない。英語「～」の意味は「約」になる。

(2) 小数点の前後

○ The medicine cost $10.25

× The medicine cost $10. 25

(3) ％と数字の間

○ Smoking is the cause of about 90% of all deaths due to lung cancer.

× Smoking is the cause of about 90 % of all deaths due to lung cancer.

(4) 略字記号としてピリオドが一つのまとまった語句の間に用いられるとき

○ a.m.   p.m.   M.A.   O.K.

× a.m.   p.m.   M.A.   O.K.

(5) スラッシュの前後

○ For healthy adults, 1 km/h is a very slow walking speed.

× For healthy adults, 1 km / h is a very slow walking speed.

95

4. イタリックを使う場合

(1) 英語以外の外国語の表現や学名

in situ   *Kokumin Kenko Hoken* (national health insurance in Japan) *Helicobacter pylori*

(2) 学術誌名、書籍のタイトル

The ALLHAT Officers and Coordinators for the ALLHAT Collaborative Research Group. Major outcomes in high-risk hypertensive patients randomized to angiotensin-converting enzyme inhibitor or calcium channel blocker vs diuretic: The Antihypertensive and Lipid-Lowering Treatment to Prevent Heart Attack Trial (ALLHAT). *JAMA*. 2002;288:2981-2997

5. 外国の人名

英語やヨーロッパの言語は、通常、名（first name/given name）から姓（last name/family name/surname）の順で表します(例：Leonard DiCaprio)。姓名の順で表記する場合、姓の後にコンマを入れることで、それが姓であると示します（例：DiCaprio, Leonard）。

B. 発表スライドの作り方のコツ

　発表用の視覚資料を作るときは、スライドに長い文を詰め込まないことが重要です。長い文は、箇条書きにして視覚的に見やすくまとめましょう。箇条書きには、特徴的なスタイルや守るべきルールがあります。見出しもなるべく短くまとめましょう。

1. 箇条書きのスタイル＆ルール

(1) 列挙する事項の品詞や文法構造を同一に揃える

(2) 主語を省くなどの省略形を用いる

(3) 全体を通して大文字、小文字の使い方は統一させる（例えばスライド3の箇条書きは全て大文字で始まっている）。

2. 参考例

　以下は高血圧についての説明文とその内容を発表用のスライドにまとめたものです。スライドを作る際に参考にしましょう。

Hypertension (high blood pressure) is a common condition that can lead to serious complications if untreated. These complications can include stroke, heart failure, heart attack, and kidney damage. Making dietary changes and losing weight are effective treatments for reducing blood pressure. Other lifestyle changes that can help to reduce blood pressure include stopping smoking, reducing stress, reducing alcohol consumption, and exercising regularly. These changes are effective when used alone but often have the greatest benefit when used together. Many patients with hypertension will also require medications to lower their blood pressure to safe levels.

Patient education: High blood pressure, diet, and weight (Beyond the Basics)
https://www.uptodate.com/contents/high-blood-pressure-diet-and-weight-beyond-the-basics
Retrieved on Jan. 29, 2018

スライド１：タイトル「高血圧と向き合う」

Dealing with Hypertension

Name:_____

Affiliation:_____

スライド２：高血圧の定義

What is hypertension?

Hypertension:
- is more commonly known as high blood pressure
- can cause serious complications
  - Stroke
  - Heart failure
  - Heart attack
  - Kidney damage

スライド３：高血圧の治療

How can hypertension be treated?
- Making dietary changes
- Losing weight
- Stopping smoking
- Reducing stress
- Reducing alcohol consumption
- Exercising regularly
- Taking medications

スライド４：参考文献

①情報源、②更新日時、③サイトの題名、④入手した日付、⑤参照したURLの順番に記載

Reference(s):

UpToDate. (2018, July 05). Patient education: High blood pressure, diet, and weight (Beyond the Basics). Retrieved on Aug. 17, 2019, from https://www.uptodate.com/contents/high-blood-pressure-diet-and-weight-beyond-the-basics

5 論文に出てくる表現集

以下は、実験系の理系論文に頻出する表現をまとめたものです。参考にしましょう。

A. 論文頻出の動詞

仮説 結果 考察	仮説を立てる、予想する	propose（提唱する）hypothesize（仮説を立てる） assume（仮定する）estimate , predict（推定・予想する）
	調べる、取り組む	examine, investigate, study, test（調べる、研究する） address（取り組む）
	示す	show, illustrate, exhibit, present, represent（示す）
	発見する	find, discover（発見する）detect（検出する） observe（観察する）isolate（分離する） identify（特定・同定する）
	明らかにする、決定する	confirm（確認する）verify, validate（検証する） clarify, reveal, uncover, elucidate（明らかにする） determine（決定する）demonstrate, prove（証明する） establish（確立する）identify（特定・同定する）
	示唆する	suggest, indicate, imply（示唆する）
実験 方法	行う、用いる	carry out, conduct, implement（実施する） perform（行う）use, employ, utilize（用いる）
	作る、開発する	create, construct, generate, prepare（作る） develop（開発する）
	分ける、選択する	separate, divide（分ける）isolate（単離する） purify（精製する）select, chose（選択する）
	処置する、受ける	treat（処置する）add（加える） receive, undergo, expose（受ける）
	計測する	measure（計測する）quantify（数量化する） quantitate（定量化する）
	分析する、評価する	analyze, assay（分析・解析する） evaluate, assess（評価する）
反応	反応する	respond, react, interact（反応する）
	生じる	emerge（現れる）arise, originate（生じる） occur, take place（起こる）
	変化させる	alter, change, convert, modify（変化させる）
	促進させる、刺激する	promote, facilitate, accelerate（促進させる） stimulate（刺激する）activate（活性化する） enhance（増強させる）
	増加する、上昇する	increase, go up, elevate, rise, jump, soar（増加・上昇する）
	減少する、下降する	decrease, go down, fall, lower, reduce, drop, decline（減少・下降する）

B. 図表の説明に用いられる表現

図	figure	表	table
題名	title, caption	凡例、説明文	legend
ラベル	label	フローチャート	flowchart
折れ線グラフ	line graph/chart	棒グラフ	bar graph/chart
円グラフ	pie graph/chart	散布図	scatter plot
X軸	X-axis, horizontal axis	Y軸	Y-axis, vertical axis
単位	unit	目盛り	scale
○●	open/closed circle	□■	open/closed square
△▲	open/closed triangle	実線	solid line
点線	dotted line	破線	broken line
列	column	行	line, row
1×10^6	one time ten to the power of six	1×10^{-6}	one time ten to the negative power of six
脚注マーク	*, †, §, ||, ¶	約10mm	~10 mm

C. 省略語・ラテン語表現

略語・表現	英語	日本語
ca.	about	約
cf.	compare	と比較せよ、参照せよ
e.g.	for example	例えば
et al.	and others	及びその他（複数の著者を示す）
etc.	and so on	など
i.e.	that is	すなわち
n	number(s)	数
N.A.	not available, not applicable	データなし
N.D.	not done, not determined, no data	データなし
vs.	versus: against	に対して
in situ	in the original place	生体内で（の）
in vitro	in artificial conditions, often in a test tube	試験管内、体外で（の）
in vivo	inside a living body	生体内で（の）
in silico	in a computer	コンピュータ内で（の）

6 発音に注意すべき単語

体の部位や症状、病名などには発音が難しいものが含まれています。また、外来語として入ってきている単語は、元になる英語と発音が異なっている場合も多いので気を付けましょう。（🔊 **Track14-1**）

Achilles' tendon*	アキレス腱	jaundice	黄疸
acne	にきび	jaw	顎
allergy	アレルギー	leukocyte	白血球
ankle**	足首	lung	肺
anus	肛門	lymph	リンパ
aorta	大動脈	meninges	髄膜
appetite	食欲	migraine	片頭痛
artery	動脈	nausea	吐き気、むかつき
blood	血	nosebleed	鼻血
breath	息	nostril	鼻腔
breathe	息をする	numb	しびれている
bronchus	気管支	obesity	肥満
cerebellum	小脳	palm	手のひら
cerebrum	大脳	paralysis	麻痺
cough	咳（をする）	patient	患者
diabetes	糖尿病	pharynx	咽頭
diaper	おむつ【米】	phlegm	痰
diaphragm	横隔膜	saliva	唾液
drowsy	眠い	sore muscle	筋肉痛
dullness	だるさ	stomach	お腹
duodenum	十二指腸	thigh	太もも
eczema	湿疹	thumb	親指
edema	むくみ	tongue	舌
embryo	胎芽	trachea	気管
erythrocyte	赤血球	tumor	腫瘍
esophagus【米】, oesophagus【英】	食道	ulcer	潰瘍
eyebrow	眉毛	urine	尿
fatigue	疲労	vena cava	大静脈
headache	頭痛	virus	ウイルス
hemorrhage	出血	womb	子宮
hormone	ホルモン	yawn	あくびをする

*人名を冠した用語の頭文字は大文字とする。例えば、Achilles' tendon のような部位、Parkinson's disease, Crohn's disease のような病名、Okazaki fragment のような物質などがある。

**uncle とは発音が違うことに注意

7 Affixで覚える専門用語

　医療系で扱う英語には、多くの専門用語が含まれます。専門用語の学習は、単語をそのまま暗記するのではなく、意味のまとまり（Affix*）に分けてそれぞれの意味を覚えましょう。そうすることで、新しい単語を見た時もAffixの知識を用いて意味を類推できます。本書で扱う英文に使われている専門用語30個に含まれるAffixを覚えましょう。

（🔊 Track14-2）

*Affixは、本書で語根、接頭辞、接尾辞をまとめて示す表現となっています。

Lesson	単語	単語和訳	Affix 1	Affix 1 和訳	Affix 2	Affix 2 和訳	Affix 3	Affix 3 和訳
L3, 9-13	angiotensin	アンジオテンシン	angi(o)-	血管	tens-	緊張	-in	(化学)物質名
L3	antifungal	抗真菌剤、抗真菌性の	ant(i)-	抗	fung(i)-	かび、真菌		
L6, 7	antihypertensive	降圧療法の	ant(i)-	反、対、抗	hyper-	過、過剰	tens-	緊張
L9-13	arterial	動脈の	arteri(o)-	動脈				
L9-13	atherosclerotic	アテローム性動脈硬化性	ather(o)-	粥状の、脂肪のかす	scler(o)-	硬化		
L3, 5, 9-13	cardiovascular	心血管の	cardi(o)-	心臓	vascul(o)-	血管		
L3	contraindication	禁忌	contra-	反、逆	indicate	薬剤の適応がある（単語）		
L9-13	coronary	冠状の、心臓の	coron(o)-	冠				
L1	diarrhea【米】, diarrhoea【英】	下痢	dia-	通して、通過	-rrhea	流出、排出、漏		
L3, 9-13	diuretic	利尿剤	dia-	通って、超えて	urin(o)-	尿	-ic	剤
L6, 9-13	dyslipidemia【米】, dyslipidaemia【英】	脂質異常症	dys-	異常	lip(i)-	脂肪	-emia	血液の状態
L9-13	gastrointestinal	消化管の	gastr(o)-	胃	intesntine	腸（単語）		
L3	haemodynamically【英】, hemodynamically【米】	血行動態的に	haem(o)-【英】, hem(o)-【米】,	血液	dynam(o)-	力		
L3	hepatic	肝臓の	hepat(o)-	肝臓				
L3	hyperglycaemia	高血糖症	hyper-	過、過剰	glyc(o)-	糖	-emia	血液の状態
L3	hypotension	低血圧	hyp(o)-	下、低	tens-	緊張		
L3	insomnia	不眠症	im-, in-	非、不	somni-	睡眠	-ia	病態
L1	intraocular	眼球内	intra-	内、内部	ocul(o)-	眼		
L3	intravenous	静脈内	intra-	内、内部	ven(o)-	静脈		

101

Lesson	単語	単語和訳	Affix 1	Affix 1 和訳	Affix 2	Affix 2 和訳	Affix 3	Affix 3 和訳
L3	lactation	乳の分泌、授乳	lact(o)-	乳				
L3	malignant	悪性	mal-	悪、不良				
L9-13	myocardial	心筋の	myo-	筋肉	cardi(o)-	心臓		
L3	pediatric[米], paediatric[英]	小児科	ped(i)-	小児	-iatric	医療（科）の、治療の		
L3	pharmacokinetics	薬物動態(学)	pharmac(o)-	薬	kinet(o)-	運動	-ics	～学
L3	pharmacotherapeutics	薬物治療学	pharmac(o)-	薬	therapeut(o)-	療法	-ics	～学
L3	pulmonary	肺の	pulmon(o)-	肺				
L3	renal	腎臓の	ren(o)-	腎臓				
L9-13	revascularization[米], revascularisation[英]	再灌流、血管再開通術	re-	再	vascul(o)-	血管、脈管		
L3	rhinitis	鼻炎	rhin(o)-	鼻	-itis	炎症		
L3	vasospastic (angina)	血管攣縮性（狭心症）	vas(o)-	血管、脈管	spasm(o)-	痙攣		

監修者紹介

野口　ジュディー（Ph.D.）
2001 年　バーミンガム大学大学院英語研究科修了
現　在　神戸学院大学　名誉教授
　　　　大阪大学大学院工学研究科　非常勤講師
　　　　大阪大学大学院医学系研究科　非常勤講師
　　　　神戸大学大学院工学研究科　非常勤講師
　　　　神戸大学大学院保健学研究科　非常勤講師

著者紹介

天ヶ瀬　葉子（Ph.D.）
2002 年　ケンブリッジ大学大学院生物学研究科薬理学専攻修了
現　在　大阪医科薬科大学薬学部　准教授
　　　　京都薬科大学　非常勤講師

スミス　朋子（Ph.D.）
2005 年　カリフォルニア大学バークレー校大学院言語学研究科修了
現　在　大阪医科薬科大学薬学部　教授

堀　朋子　修士（言語文化学）
2007 年　大阪外国語大学大学院地域言語社会研究科通訳翻訳専修コース修了
現　在　大阪医科薬科大学　非常勤講師

神前　陽子（Ed.D.）
2006 年　テンプル大学大学院英語教授法研究科修了
現　在　武庫川女子大学薬学部　非常勤講師
　　　　大阪医科薬科大学　非常勤講師
　　　　神戸大学大学院理学研究科　非常勤講師
　　　　テンプル大学応用言語学博士課程　非常勤講師

玉巻　欣子（Ph.D.）
1990 年　ニューヨーク州立大学ストーニーブルック校言語学部修了
2013 年　神戸大学大学院医学研究科医科学専攻修了
現　在　神戸薬科大学　教授

村木　美紀子　修士
2002 年　ハーバード大学公衆衛生大学院医療政策経営学専攻修了
現　在　大阪医科薬科大学　非常勤講師
　　　　摂南大学　非常勤講師

NDC491　　111p　　26cm

これからの薬学英語

2019 年 9 月 30 日　第 1 刷発行
2025 年 7 月 11 日　第 11 刷発行

監修者　野口ジュディー
著　者　天ヶ瀬葉子・神前陽子・スミス朋子・玉巻欣子・堀朋子・村木美紀子
発行者　篠木和久
発行所　株式会社　講談社
　　　　〒 112-8001　東京都文京区音羽 2-12-21
　　　　　　販　売　(03) 5395-5817
　　　　　　業　務　(03) 5395-3615

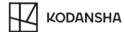

編　集　株式会社　講談社サイエンティフィク
　　　　代表　堀越俊一
　　　　〒 162-0825　東京都新宿区神楽坂 2-14　ノービィビル
　　　　　　編　集　(03) 3235-3701
本文データ制作　株式会社エヌ・オフィス
印刷・製本　株式会社ＫＰＳプロダクツ

落丁本・乱丁本は購入書店名を明記のうえ，講談社業務宛にお送りください．送料小社負担にてお取替えします．なお，この本の内容についてのお問い合わせは，講談社サイエンティフィク宛にお願いいたします．定価はカバーに表示してあります．

© J. Noguchi, Y. Amagase, Y. Kozaki, T. Smith, K. Tamamaki, T. Hori and M. Muraki, 2019

本書のコピー，スキャン，デジタル化等の無断複製は著作権法上での例外を除き禁じられています．本書を代行業者等の第三者に依頼してスキャンやデジタル化することはたとえ個人や家庭内の利用でも著作権法違反です．

Printed in Japan

ISBN978-4-06-517253-7